The CBD DOG BISCUIT COOKBOOK

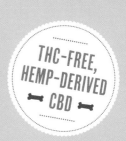

paw cbd™

THC-FREE, HEMP-DERIVED CBD

HUMAN TESTED
ANIMAL APPROVED

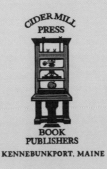

CIDER MILL PRESS

BOOK PUBLISHERS

KENNEBUNKPORT, MAINE

13-Digit ISBN: 978-1-64643-227-1
10-Digit ISBN: 1-64643-227-4

This book may be ordered by mail from the publisher. Please include $4.95 for postage and handling. Please support your local bookseller first!

Books published by Cider Mill Press Book Publishers are available at special discounts for bulk purchases in the United States by corporations, institutions, and other organizations. For more information, please contact the publisher.

Cider Mill Press Book Publishers
"Where good books are ready for press"
12 Spring Street
PO Box 454
Kennebunkport, Maine 04046

Visit us online
cidermillpress.com

Printed in China

1 2 3 4 5 6 7 8 9 0
First Edition

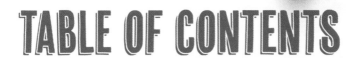

TABLE OF CONTENTS

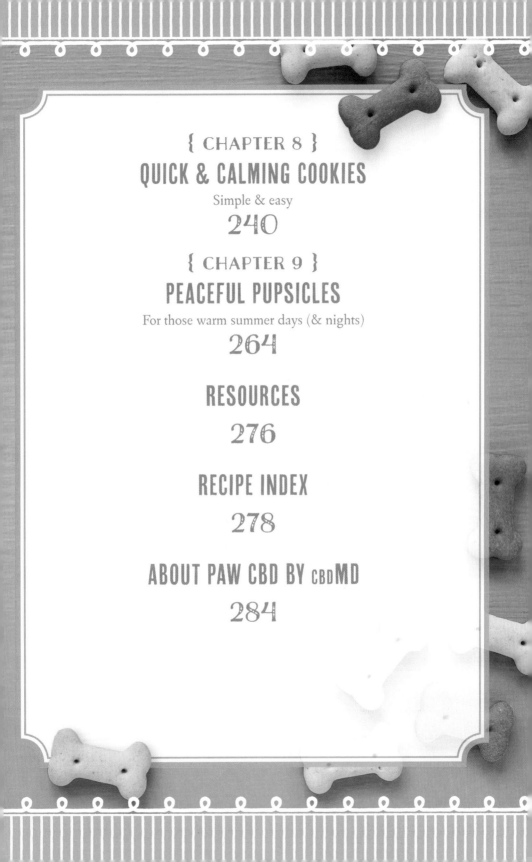

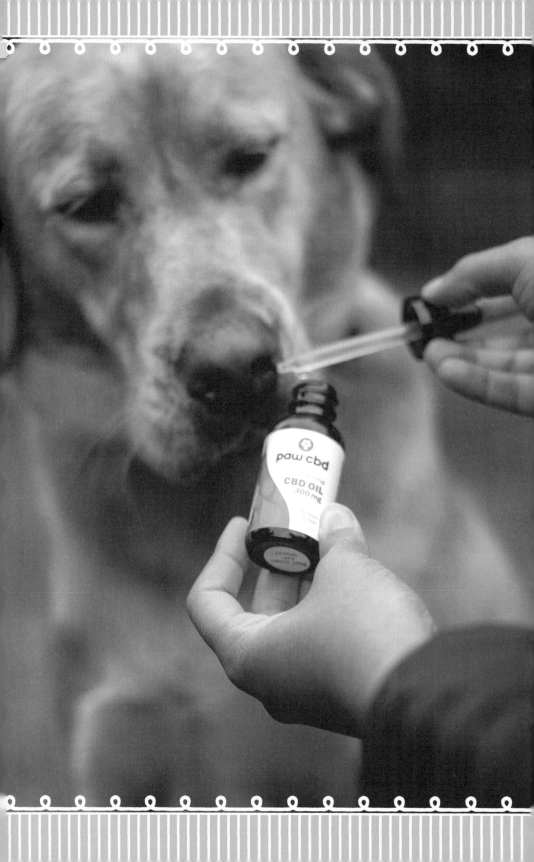

INTRODUCTION

If you don't already use CBD yourself, you probably know people who do. Your workout buddy recommends it for post activity recovery, or your stressed-out coworkers say it helps them relax. Or your sister swears by it for better sleep, and even your parents (or grandparents!) might agree that it's great for easing their aching knees and joints.

Even without firsthand experience, most of us are aware that CBD is growing in popularity and quickly becoming part of everyday lives and wellness routines. With so many people using CBD and finding positive results, it's no wonder, then, that they are increasingly interested in sharing those benefits with their pets. And while it can be beneficial for most pets, CBD for dogs is becoming especially popular.

But, as with any trend, it's important to be informed. Your dog can't speak for itself, so you have a lot of responsibility to educate yourself as a pet parent before introducing something new to your pup's lifestyle. Before you put on your apron and pull out the mixing bowls, here are a few things you should know about making dog treats with CBD oil.

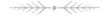

{ WHAT IS CBD? }

First, let's answer the most basic question: What is CBD oil? While it's easy to get into a very detailed discussion of CBD facts, the simple answer to this question is that CBD oil is made from CBD, or cannabidiol, an active ingredient found in both the hemp and the marijuana plant. Hemp is a very specific type of cannabis plant that is different from marijuana cannabis because of its extremely low concentration of THC. Industrial hemp plants, to be labeled as such, cannot contain more than 0.3% THC.

THC, or tetrahydrocannabinol, is a chemical compound extracted from the cannabis plant. It causes the psychoactive effects that people understand as getting "high" from marijuana. But the cannabis plant has more than 80 different chemical compounds besides THC—one of which is CBD. This means that CBD oil is not psychoactive and will not get you (or your pet!) "high" or "buzzed" or any of the things associated with marijuana.

CBD oil is simply CBD that has been pulled from the plant and diffused into a carrier oil for better application and consumption. Most carrier oils are natural, including MCT (coconut-based) oil and hemp seed oil.

Much of this detail was outlined in the 2018 Farm Bill, which legalized broad cultivation of the hemp plant. The important thing to know as a pet owner is that hemp-derived CBD products for dogs are legal and can benefit your pet in a myriad of ways.

{ CBD FOR DOGS }

CBD offers overall wellness support for both people and pets. Because dogs and humans (and all mammals) have an endocannabinoid system (ECS), CBD can positively affect those bodily systems in many of the same ways. The ECS first became the focus of research in the '90s, and scientists are still studying its complexity. However, it's become clear that this system affects a variety of processes in the body, including (but not limited to) sleep, stress, mood, appetite, and digestion.

CBD may offer several benefits, like supporting a sense of calm, helping manage signs of daily stress, and complementing a pet's regular wellness routine. A multitude of happy pet owners who have given their dogs CBD reported good results for common concerns such as:

• Noise aversion (storms, fireworks)
• Separation issues or stressful situations
• Overall health and wellness
• Active lifestyle support and maintenance
• Mobility support (joint or age-related stiffness)

Every dog is different, and results may vary, but the ability to adjust serving sizes to fit the needs of your particular pooch is one of the best things about CBD. And, of course, it is always recommended that you consult your veterinarian, especially if you have concerns about your pet's unique health or behavior issues.

{ IS CBD SAFE FOR DOGS? }

While you might have many questions about CBD for pets, "Is CBD safe?" is the most common. The short answer? Yes, CBD is generally regarded as safe for dogs to take. If it is properly sourced, manufactured, and third-party tested, then your dog should be able to use CBD without issues. But buyer beware. With so many pet CBD products flooding the market, it's essential to do your research, because not all products are made the same.

{ CHOOSING THE RIGHT CBD PRODUCT }

To ensure you're getting the best product for your dog, you'll need to understand how CBD oil is made. The extraction process impacts the quality of the final product. There are two primary ways to extract CBD oil from an industrial hemp plant: ethanol extraction and CO_2 extraction.

Ethanol extraction uses ethanol, a high-grade grain alcohol, to separate CBD from the plant itself. This method is incredibly consistent and stable; it can be done in many different conditions without threat to the quality of the final product. This is not as true of CO_2 extraction, which strips the plant of CBD using very, very cold CO_2. The low temperatures of this extraction process make it a little more volatile, though the final product can be extremely pure when done correctly.

Perhaps more important than the extraction process is the type of CBD that is used. CBD products can be made using:

• **CBD ISOLATE**, which is only pure, isolated CBD. These products, while appropriate for some, can leave behind useful terpenes and cannabinoids in the hemp plant that can increase the benefits of CBD.

- **FULL-SPECTRUM CBD** features all the compounds in the plant, including some traces of THC.
- **BROAD-SPECTRUM CBD** is a sort of in-between that includes many of the plant's compounds but removes THC molecules.

When buying CBD for your pet, you should know the answers to these questions to make sure you're getting a safe, effective product:

- **WHERE IS THE HEMP GROWN, AND HOW?**
  The United States has pretty intense rules about farming hemp on American soil. So with domestically grown hemp, you can rest assured that your CBD pet product was derived from a healthy, safe plant.
- **ARE ALL INGREDIENTS CLEARLY LISTED WITH NO FILLERS OR ANYTHING ARTIFICIAL INCLUDED?**
- **IS IT MADE WITH PREMIUM, HEMP-DERIVED CBD?**
- **DOES THE PRODUCT INDICATE IT HAS BEEN THIRD-PARTY LAB TESTED TO BE FREE OF THC?**
  A trustworthy product will have a Certificate of Analysis from a third-party laboratory that ensures it is free of THC.
- **IS IT SPECIALLY FORMULATED FOR YOUR PET'S SAFETY?**
  While it might be tempting to use the same CBD oil you have for yourself, anything you give your pets should be made specifically for them with only pure, safe ingredients.
- **DOES IT COME IN STRENGTHS BASED ON YOUR PET'S WEIGHT?**
- **ARE SERVING SUGGESTIONS AND DIRECTIONS CLEAR?**

If you educate yourself on what to look for, you can be confident in giving your pet CBD. Of course, it's always best to consult your veterinarian before starting a regular CBD routine for your pet.

{ POTENTIAL CBD SIDE EFFECTS }

Because so few studies have been done on CBD for pets specifically, there is not much research yet exploring the side effects of CBD oil in dogs. However, CBD oil for dogs has now been on the market long enough that any negative side effects would most likely have been reported and addressed at this point.

What we do know is that, in people, a few minor side effects have been noted at higher doses, so watch your dog closely for any of the following:

- **DROWSINESS:** Many dog owners use CBD for its calming effect, but it can sometimes cause drowsiness if too much is given.
- **DRY MOUTH:** Because it can decrease saliva production, look for signs of increased thirst in your dog when giving them CBD.
- **LOWERED BLOOD PRESSURE:** In people, large amounts of CBD can temporarily bring down blood pressure, causing brief light-headedness. While this may not affect dogs in the same way, it's always best to monitor your dog when giving them CBD.

{ HOW MUCH CBD OIL TO USE }

Once you've chosen the best product for your purposes, you'll need to decide how much CBD to give to your dog. Serving size is a significant part of introducing CBD to your pet for the first time.

CBD oil products for dogs will come in different strengths and serving sizes, and how much you give to your pet will depend on their weight. Here are some steps for introducing this new product to your pet:

1. Read the packaging and instructions to determine the recommended strength and serving size for your dog.
2. Talk to your veterinarian about your plans.
3. Start with the smallest recommended serving size and stick with it for 30 days. It can take time to see the benefits of CBD for dogs, so watch your pet closely for changes in activity and behavior during this time.
4. Increase the serving size by a small amount after the initial 30 days if you haven't seen the benefits.

Just like people, every dog is different, and will respond differently to CBD. Some might respond right away, while others might need more time. You know your dog best, so just keep an eye on them and then adjust the CBD strength or serving size accordingly.

As for using CBD in recipes, how much to add will depend on a few factors. First is how your dog responds to CBD. Second is the amount (mg) of CBD in the product you use. And last is the number of treats each recipe makes.

Start with the mg strength you find most effective for your dog and then decide how many treats you want to make. Then decide how much CBD per treat you want your dog to have, keeping in mind their total recommended daily serving and if you will be using the treats in combination with other daily CBD. Once you know that, add the appropriate amount to the recipe.

When using CBD oil in recipes, carefully follow the suggested serving amounts on the CBD oil packaging, which should clearly list how many milligrams of CBD is in each serving size, not just in the whole product. Then do your math based on the overall recipe to add the appropriate amount.

Weight of dog in lbs.	Suggested mg of CBD per day
Under 25 lbs.	5mg
25–50 lbs.	10mg
51–75 lbs.	25mg
76–99 lbs.	50mg
100+ lbs.	100mg

For your convenience, a bookmark with this table can be found at the back of this book. If you ever use a recipe that does not specifically list the amount of CBD oil to use, use this simple formula: Total recipe servings x desired amount of CBD per serving = total amount of CBD used for the recipe. For example, if a recipe makes 8 servings and you want each one to contain 10mg of CBD, you'll need to use 80mg of CBD.

NOTE: If your dog is already using CBD and you also want to give them treats, just be sure that you are not giving your dog more than the daily recommended mg of CBD for their size between delivery methods.

{ BAKING WITH CBD OIL }

The details of cooking with CBD oil depend partly on what oil is used as the medium for the CBD. Look for CBD that uses MCT oil, which is good for low- to mid-temperature cooking. If you're making baked dog treats with CBD oil, it's ideal to keep the baking temperature at or below 350°F to maintain its potency.

Note that since CBD oil can be sensitive to heat and light, you should always store any leftover baked goods in an airtight container in a cool, dark place or in the refrigerator. Most recipes will be good for up to one week unless otherwise indicated.

When baking, you can add a little extra-special touch by using different flavors of CBD oil in your CBD dog treat recipes. Get creative with the flavor your canine companion loves best!

SUBSTITUTIONS

A common substitution is the replacement of eggs in any of the recipes. If your dog is allergic to eggs, here are some substitutions you can try:

1 MEDIUM TO SMALL BANANA = 1 EGG
3 TABLESPOONS APPLESAUCE (USE UNSWEETENED) = 1 EGG

But please keep in mind that they will not cook exactly the same way an egg would, so add the liquid portion of the recipe slowly, since it may require using more or less due to the difference in moisture these substitutes add.

Another common substitution people look for is different flour options. We choose to use a combination of organic oat flour and organic brown rice flour. All these recipes are wheat, corn, and soy free, and we recommend you use a wheat-free flour if you have the opportunity, as wheat is such a common dog allergy these days. When you swap a flour in the recipes with one of these or another one you have purchased, use the same amount of total flour that the recipe calls for, but add the liquid portion slowly, since the flour may absorb more or less moisture due to the substitution. Flour can hold up to 40% of its weight in moisture, so humidity or lack thereof can greatly affect the amount of liquid your recipe needs to come together to a usable consistency.

YIELDS

We tried to make these recipes as simple as possible and recommend using whatever you have on hand to form the shapes of the treats. That said, we cannot state precisely how many treats each recipe will make. We also don't know your intended audience. If you have a Chihuahua, you'll obviously want to make smaller-sized treats (they'll also cook faster, so keep an eye on them). And if a Great Dane is your canine companion, make them larger (again, watch them, because they might need a little longer to cook). Most of the recipes are about the same size, so once you make one, you can anticipate how many treats you'll get out of any of them. Using a standard 3" or so cookie cutter, you can estimate a yield of 20 to 30 treats per batch and a little over one pound of treats.

SOFT OR CRUNCHY?

You know your dog and their tastes or dietary needs. If you want the treats to be softer, cook them a little less or at a lower heat (definitely keep them in the refrigerator too). If you want your treats to be a little harder, cook them longer at a lower heat. Or, when they are finished cooking, turn the oven off but leave them in there on the tray to cool for a few hours or overnight.

STORAGE TIPS

Remember that these recipes are all for homemade, preservative-free treats. With that in mind, they can't sit out the way processed dog treats can. We recommend storing them in a plastic bag or container in the refrigerator. Even in there they will still get moldy, like your leftovers, so store only an amount you think you will use within a week. Any extras (since these recipes yield more than a week's worth of treats for most households) can be frozen to thaw out later (this works great) or given away as gifts to your friends, neighbors, or coworkers.

If you are looking to keep the treats on the counter, in your pocket for training, etc., and want them to stay fresh for your pup, you will need to make sure you cook them nice and crispy. Thinner is better for this. If the cookies are cut thinner, they will cook more quickly and get crispier, allowing them to stay fresh longer without refrigeration. Add a few more minutes to your cook time to make sure they are crispy, and allow them to cool and air out overnight, to really ensure the moisture is out of them before you move them to another container. Again, please keep in mind that we cannot know what the moisture levels are in the treats you make yourself; therefore, we cannot tell you a specific amount of time they can maintain freshness out of the fridge. But a general rule of thumb is thinner is better, crispier is necessary, and it's safer to stay with the nonmeaty recipes for this purpose.

{ LET'S GET STARTED }

At the end of the day, we all want our pets to be and feel their best. Whether you share your life with an active adventure dog, a loveable couch-potato pooch, or a canine companion that falls somewhere in between, CBD might be the perfect addition to their daily routine. Treats make a great choice for portability and consistent delivery (meaning the exact same serving size every time).

You'll be surprised at how easy it is to make CBD dog treats at home. Let's get started with tasty, tail-wagging recipes that are fun to make and will have your best friend sitting up and begging for more!

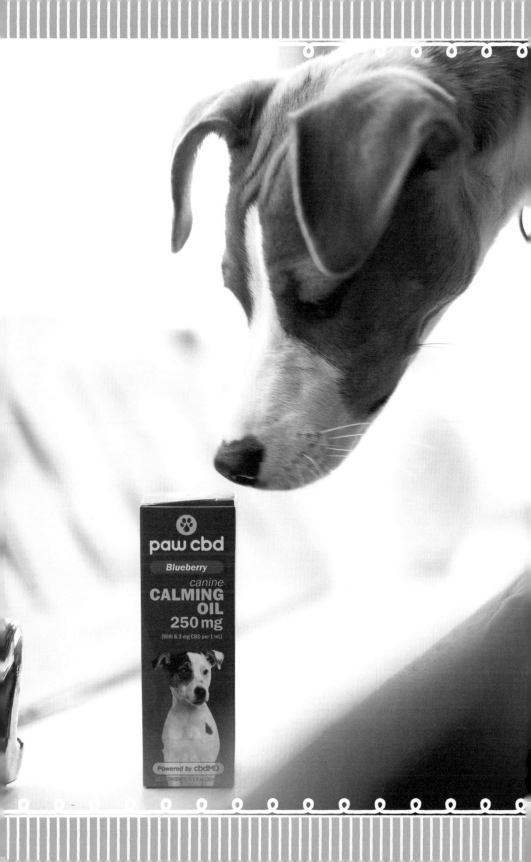

CHAPTER 1

RELAXATION CELEBRATION

A special treat for your favorite four-legger for each month of the year

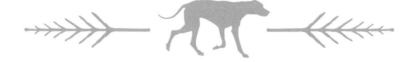

Life without celebrations would be no fun at all, right? Dogs are lucky in that they need nothing more than our very presence to find cause for celebration. And occasions marked with yummy treats soon become particularly special for them. Still, large gatherings and family traditions—from feasts to fireworks—can be a source of stress for our canine companions. These recipes will help them relax and enjoy the festivities, with safe options that allow your dog to celebrate every exciting event with you.

When all is said and done, if there is an event worth celebrating with family and friends, there's no reason not to include something special for your four-legged family member. Here are 12 recipes to correspond with a significant celebration in every month of the year.

Choose to use organic ingredients in these recipes, like we do!

HALF & HALF COOKIES

Usher in the New Year on the right paw. If you're staying home and enjoying a festive dinner with family and friends, consider going black tie to transform the evening into a memorable, formal affair. Dogs look great with their tuxes and tails on too, and when they greet your guests at the door rocking a black bow tie or tiara, everyone will know there's a party goin' on. Watch that your guests don't go for these scrumptious-looking black-and-white cookies; they'll be tempted!

FOR THE DOUGH:

1 ½ c. oat flour

1 ½ c. brown rice flour

½ c. peanut butter (unsalted)

1 tbsp. honey

1 egg

CBD oil (see page 16 for dosage amounts)

½ c. water (add slowly)

FOR THE TOPPING:

8 oz. white chocolate chips (these are safe for dogs)

8 oz. carob chips (do NOT substitute with chocolate)

Preheat oven to 350°F. Combine all dough ingredients (except the water) together. Add water slowly and mix until a dough forms (if too dry, add more water; too wet, add a bit more flour). You may not need all the water if you reach a good consistency first. Roll out on a lightly floured surface to ¼" thickness. Use a round cookie cutter or the rim of an upside-down glass to cut out 2" circles in the dough. Line a cookie sheet with parchment paper (for easy cleanup), and place the cookies on the sheet (they can be rather close together, as they don't grow much while cooking).

Bake 20 to 25 minutes or until golden brown. Transfer and let cool completely on a wire rack.

When the cookies are cooling, prepare the topping. To do so, heat the white chocolate chips over low heat in a double boiler or in the microwave until melted. Dip half of each cookie into the melted white chocolate and place back on a wire rack to cool. Once all cookies are cooled, at least to the touch, heat the carob chips in a double boiler or in the microwave until melted. Dip the other half of each cookie into the melted carob and place back on a wire rack to cool.

Store the cookies in an airtight container in the refrigerator. For more options, read the "Storage Tips" section on page 19.

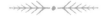

BE MINE, VALENTINE

At this time of year, when it's appropriate to go over the top in displaying your affection, go ahead and really shower it on your dog. With these healthy, red-colored, heart-shaped cookies, you can spoil them knowing you won't be plying them with a lot of artificial ingredients. Natural food colorings are made from plants and vegetables and are readily available in any health food store or online.

1 ½ c. oat flour

1 ½ c. brown rice flour

½ c. grated Parmesan cheese

6-oz. can tomato paste

1 tsp. basil

1 egg

CBD oil (see page 16 for dosage amounts)

½ c. water (add slowly)

Natural red food coloring (optional)

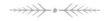

Preheat oven to 350°F. Combine all dough ingredients (except the water) together. Add enough red food coloring to reach the desired color. Add water slowly and mix until a dough forms (if too dry, add more water; too wet, add a bit more flour). You may not need all the water if you reach a good consistency first. Roll out on a lightly floured surface to ¼" thickness. Use a heart-shaped cookie cutter (or a knife) to cut out shapes. Line a cookie sheet with parchment paper (for easy cleanup), and place the cookies on the sheet (they can be rather close together, as they don't grow much while cooking).

Bake 20 to 25 minutes or until golden brown. Transfer and let cool completely on a wire rack. Store the cookies in an airtight container in the refrigerator. For more options, read the "Storage Tips" section on page 19.

NATURAL FOOD COLORINGS

Beets are the source of a lot of the red natural food colorants. You can change the color of the dough with these other natural colorants for other occasions. Remember, though, that these fruits and vegetables add flavor too. Use sparingly to be sure your dog will like it and so you don't overpower the other flavors. Also, never use coffee or any kind of grape juice to add color (or flavor) to a recipe, as these ingredients are harmful to dogs.

BLUEISH-PURPLE: Blueberries, Red Cabbage
PURPLE: Blackberries
RED: Beets, Tomatoes
PINKISH-RED: Beets, Strawberries, Hibiscus
GREEN: Spinach, Kale
YELLOWISH-ORANGE: Turmeric, Curry Powder
ORANGE: Annatto

POT OF GOLD

On St. Patrick's Day—March 17—everyone is Irish for the day. Your preferred method of celebration may be to have a green bagel or beer. We don't recommend that you share that particular tradition with your dog, but you can be assured they'll stay close by your bar stool if you have a plate of these with you. And you know what? They taste pretty good with beer, so you may want to nibble on them too.

1 $^1/_2$ c. oat flour

1 $^1/_2$ c. brown rice flour

1 $^1/_2$ c. tightly packed spinach leaves

$^1/_2$ c. shredded cheddar cheese

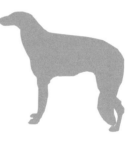

$^1/_2$ c. grated Parmesan cheese

2 tbsp. rosemary

$^1/_2$ c. oat bran

1 egg

CBD oil (see page 16 for dosage amounts)

$^1/_2$ c. water (add slowly)

Preheat oven to 350°F. Puree the spinach leaves in a food processor until smooth. Combine all ingredients (except the water) together. Add water slowly and mix until a dough forms (if too dry, add more water; too wet, add a bit more flour). You may not need all the water if you reach a good consistency first. Roll out on a lightly floured surface to ¼" thickness. Use a shamrock-shaped cookie cutter (or a knife) to cut out shapes. Line a cookie sheet with parchment paper (for easy cleanup), and place the cookies on the sheet (they can be rather close together, as they don't grow much while cooking).

Bake 20 to 25 minutes or until golden brown. Transfer and let cool completely on a wire rack. Store the cookies in an airtight container in the refrigerator. For more options, read the "Storage Tips" section on page 19.

ROSEMARY

Rosemary is an excellent antioxidant and full of vitamin C, vitamin A, iron, folic acid, dietary fiber, and potassium. It is a natural antibiotic and antiseptic and is known to have anti-inflammatory, antiallergic, and antifungal properties. It supports immune system functions and defends against free radical damage.

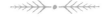

SOME-BUNNY TO LOVE

For all you hound people out there, you know the thrill that the mention of the Easter Bunny brings for many of your dogs. Is there anything better than ol' Peter Cottontail's fresh scent in the hedgerow? Well, for those deprived of the Real Thing, these treats will surely come in a close second; in fact, they may even keep your super-sniffer away from the stash of goodies you're trying to hide from you-know-who. While you're making these, remember, spring is just around the corner!

FOR THE CAKE:

2 c. pureed carrots

2 ½ c. oat flour

3 eggs

½ c. honey

2 tsp. baking powder

½ tsp. baking soda

1 tsp. cinnamon

¼ c. safflower oil

1 tsp. vanilla

CBD oil (see page 16 for dosage amounts)

FOR THE FROSTING:

8-oz. package low-fat cream cheese (at room temperature)

2 tbsp. honey

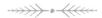

Preheat oven to 350°F. Peel and dice the carrots, then puree the carrot pieces in a food processor.

Combine the carrots with all the other ingredients in a large bowl and mix thoroughly. Place cupcake papers in a mini muffin pan (or a regular muffin pan). Spoon the mixture evenly into the papers, filling close to the top (the mix will not rise very much).

Bake 10 to 15 minutes if using the mini muffin pan or 20 to 25 minutes if using a regular-sized muffin pan. Cupcakes are done when a toothpick inserted in the center comes out clean. Let cool completely on a wire rack.

Combine frosting ingredients together and whip until well mixed and fluffy. Decorate the cupcakes. Store the cupcakes in an airtight container in the refrigerator. For more options, read the "Storage Tips" section on page 19. For more icing options, view the other icing recipes on pages 171 and 173.

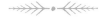

SUN'S OUT, FUN'S OUT

The days are getting longer and warmer; the flowers are blooming; spring has sprung. Celebrate the joy of a new season with these special cookies, infused with a healthy dose of sunflower seeds, cranberries, and oats—how perfect!

1 $\frac{1}{4}$ c. oat flour

1 $\frac{1}{4}$ c. brown rice flour

1 c. hulled sunflower seeds (unsalted)

$\frac{1}{2}$ c. rolled oats (the old-fashioned kind, not instant)

$\frac{1}{2}$ c. dried cranberries

$\frac{1}{4}$ c. honey

3 tbsp. applesauce (unsweetened)

1 egg

CBD oil (see page 16 for dosage amounts)

$\frac{1}{2}$ c. water (add slowly)

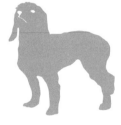

Preheat oven to 350°F. Set aside ½ c. sunflower seeds to use for topping. Combine all other ingredients (except the water) together. Add water slowly and mix until a dough forms (if too dry, add more water; too wet, add a bit more flour). You may not need all the water if you reach a good consistency first. Roll out on a lightly floured surface to ¼" thickness. Use a flower-shaped cookie cutter (or a knife) to cut into shapes. Line a cookie sheet with parchment paper (for easy cleanup), and place the cookies on the sheet (they can be rather close together, as they don't grow much while cooking).

Bake 20 to 25 minutes or until golden brown. Transfer and let cool completely on a wire rack. Store the cookies in an airtight container in the refrigerator. For more options, read the "Storage Tips" section on page 19.

OATS

Oats contain a higher concentration of protein, calcium, iron, magnesium, zinc, copper, manganese, thiamine, folacin, and vitamin E than any other unfortified whole grain (such as wheat, barley, corn, etc.). They are high in fiber, amino acids, and lipids, which contain a good balance of essential fatty acids for overall good health. Oats are a grain with a low gluten content. They have been shown to lower cholesterol and reduce the risk of heart disease.

COOKOUT COOKIES

Get out the barbeque, summertime is here! While you're enjoying classic summer dishes like BBQ chicken, ribs, sausages, and burgers paired with potato salad and other goodies, it just wouldn't be right not to have something equally scrumptious and appropriate for your dog. These cookies are like cheeseburgers with all the fixings—including a dose of healthy sesame seeds and parsley (in fact, you may want to try adding these to your burgers!).

$\frac{1}{2}$ c. lean ground beef (precooked and drained)

1 $\frac{1}{2}$ c. oat flour

1 $\frac{1}{2}$ c. potato flour

$\frac{1}{2}$ c. shredded low-fat cheddar cheese

6-oz. can tomato paste

1 tbsp. dried parsley

1 egg

CBD oil (see page 16 for dosage amounts)

$\frac{1}{2}$ c. water (add slowly)

2 tbsp. sesame seeds (save for topping)

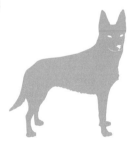

Preheat oven to 350°F. Cook and drain ground beef. Combine all ingredients (except the water and sesame seeds) together. Add water slowly and mix until a dough forms (if too dry, add more water; too wet, add a bit more flour). You may not need all the water if you reach a good consistency first. Form into hamburger-shaped patties (about 2" in diameter). Line a cookie sheet with parchment paper (for easy cleanup), and place the cookies on the sheet (they can be rather close together, as they don't grow much while cooking). Sprinkle them with the sesame seeds.

Bake 22 to 27 minutes or until golden brown. Transfer and let cool completely on a wire rack. Store the cookies in an airtight container in the refrigerator. For more options, read the "Storage Tips" section on page 19.

PARSLEY

Parsley's role as an attractive garnish has long since been replaced by that of a nutritious and delicious health benefit. Parsley is loaded with vitamins A, B, C, and K and the minerals calcium, potassium, iron, magnesium, and phosphorous, as well as protein. It is high in chlorophyll, which gives it the natural freshening power associated with combating foul-smelling breath. All these things make it a great addition to a dog's diet.

STAR-SPANGLED BISCUITS

It's fun to make a cake that looks like the American flag with strawberries and blueberries on the 4th of July, but these sensational fruits can—and should—be enjoyed all month. Their benefits are available for your dog too in these fruit-filled, naturally sweetened cookies.

1/2 c. strawberries (fresh or frozen)
1/2 c. blueberries (fresh or frozen)
1 1/4 c. oat flour
1 1/4 c. brown rice flour
1/2 c. oat bran
2 tbsp. honey
1 tsp. cinnamon
1 egg
CBD oil (see page 16 for dosage amounts)
1/4 c. water (add slowly)

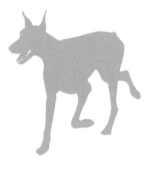

Preheat oven to 350°F. Puree strawberries and blueberries in a food processor. Combine all ingredients (except the water) together. Add water slowly and mix until a dough forms (if too dry, add more water; too wet, add a bit more flour). You may not need all the water if you reach a good consistency first. Roll out on a lightly floured surface to ¼" thickness. Use any fun patriotic-shaped cookie cutter (or a knife) to cut into shapes. Line a cookie sheet with parchment paper (for easy cleanup), and place the cookies on the sheet (they can be rather close together, as they don't grow much while cooking).

Bake 20 to 25 minutes or until golden brown. Transfer and let cool completely on a wire rack. Store the cookies in an airtight container in the refrigerator. For more options, read the "Storage Tips" section on page 19.

BERRIES

Several of the recipes in this chapter call for various berries, including cranberries, blueberries, and strawberries. Wonder no longer; all are safe for dogs. Berries are natural antioxidants; in fact, recent studies have shown that blueberries are especially rich in them. Cranberries are known for relieving urinary tract infections and promoting uterine health. Berries also contain lots of vitamin C. They are naturally sweet and tasty, and dogs really enjoy them. They can be served fresh, frozen, or dried.

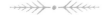

SUMMER SNACKS

Did you know that late July through mid-August are considered the "dog days of summer"? Well, let's break the heat with these tasty BBQ biscuits that your dog will be sure to go crazy for. With all those barbecues in full swing, why not treat your favorite four-legged friend to their very own chicken treat?

1 $\frac{1}{4}$ c. oat flour

1 $\frac{1}{4}$ c. brown rice flour

$\frac{1}{2}$ c. ground chicken (precooked)

$\frac{1}{2}$ c. oat bran

1 tbsp. blackstrap molasses

2 tbsp. tomato paste

1 tsp. apple cider vinegar

1 egg

CBD oil (see page 16 for dosage amounts)

$\frac{1}{2}$ c. water (add slowly)

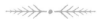

Preheat oven to 350°F. Combine all ingredients (except the water) together. Add water slowly and mix until a dough forms (if too dry, add more water; too wet, add a bit more flour). You may not need all the water if you reach a good consistency first. Roll out on a lightly floured surface to ¼" thickness. Use any shaped cookie cutter (or a knife) to cut into shapes. Line a cookie sheet with parchment paper (for easy cleanup), and place the cookies on the sheet (they can be rather close together, as they don't grow much while cooking).

Bake 25 to 30 minutes or until golden brown. Transfer and let cool completely on a wire rack. Store the cookies in an airtight container in the refrigerator. For more options, read the "Storage Tips" section on page 19.

AVOID THE ONIONS

We rely on onions to add flavor to many of our summer favorites, and it's often included in BBQ sauces. They don't harm us (though raw onions make for bad breath), but they have been shown to cause damage to dogs' red blood cells, which can lead to anemia. It's best to avoid all forms of onion in the food you give your dog—raw, cooked, and even powdered onion.

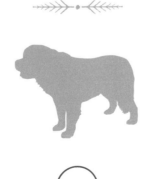

FLAVORFUL FALL TREATS

Apples are wonderful for everyone, dogs included! There's nothing like a crisp, juicy apple to signal the beginning of fall. You can feed your dog pieces of raw apple as a snack (they love to crunch them just like we do), or cook the apples down into a soft sauce (no sugar!) and add a spoonful or two to their meals. This recipe brings out the great flavor of apples with some cheddar cheese and honey—a recipe no dog can resist!

1 ½ c. oat flour

1 ½ c. brown rice flour

1 tsp. cinnamon

1 c. applesauce (unsweetened)

½ c. rolled oats (the old-fashioned kind, not instant)

1 tbsp. honey

1 egg

CBD oil (see page 16 for dosage amounts)

½ c. water (add slowly)

Preheat oven to 350°F. Combine all ingredients (except the water) together. Add water slowly and mix until a dough forms (if too dry, add more water; too wet, add a bit more flour). You may not need all the water if you reach a good consistency first. Roll out on a lightly floured surface to ¼" thickness. Use an apple-shaped cookie cutter (or a knife) to cut into shapes. Line a cookie sheet with parchment paper (for easy cleanup), and place the cookies on the sheet (they can be rather close together, as they don't grow much while cooking).

Bake 20 to 25 minutes or until golden brown. Transfer and let cool completely on a wire rack. Store the cookies in an airtight container in the refrigerator. For more options, read the "Storage Tips" section on page 19.

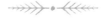

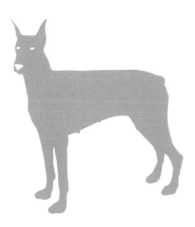

JACK-O'-LANTERN JAMBOREE

As you're preparing costumes for yourself, your kids, and your dog for the magical day of Halloween, look for recipes that include pumpkin—that super-nutritious vegetable that is the centerpiece of so many Halloween and fall celebrations. For yourself and your family, make a pumpkin soup or pumpkin bread. For your dog, make these pumpkin bites. With your tummies full, you'll be ready to turn your attention to carving the most glorious pumpkins.

1 ½ c. oat flour
1 ½ c. brown rice flour
½ c. pumpkin (canned or fresh)
2 tbsp. molasses (regular or blackstrap)
1 tsp. cinnamon
1 tsp. ground ginger
1 tbsp. honey
1 egg
CBD oil (see page 16 for dosage amounts)
½ c. water (add slowly)

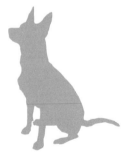

Preheat oven to 350°F. Combine all ingredients (except the water) together. Add water slowly and mix until a dough forms (if too dry, add more water; too wet, add a bit more flour). You may not need all the water if you reach a good consistency first. Roll out on a lightly floured surface to 1/4" thickness. Use a pumpkin-shaped cookie cutter (or a knife) to cut into shapes. Line a cookie sheet with parchment paper (for easy cleanup), and place the cookies on the sheet (they can be rather close together, as they don't grow much while cooking).

Bake 22 to 27 minutes or until golden brown. Transfer and let cool completely on a wire rack. Store the cookies in an airtight container in the refrigerator. For more options, read the "Storage Tips" section on page 19.

PUMPKIN, YAMS, SWEET POTATOES

Sweet potatoes and yams are high in potassium and beta-carotene (a natural antioxidant) and low in calories. They are also soothing for an upset stomach. Did you know that a tablespoon of canned or fresh sweet potatoes, yams, or pumpkin on top of your dog's food will help to regulate an upset stomach?

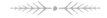

FEAST FRENZY

This is our favorite time of the year, and as the big Thanksgiving feast is being prepared, dogs get excited too. They see lots of food being made, family and friends getting together, tables being set for a special feast—and they want to share in the good times and good eats. Save the fatty gravy and skins that can lead to digestive upset in dogs for yourself (and maybe give that a little consideration too), and make these treats instead, which are like a Thanksgiving meal in a cookie—irresistible, and healthy.

$^1/_2$ c. pureed carrots
$^1/_2$ c. cooked, mashed sweet potatoes (or yams)
1 $^1/_2$ c. oat flour
1 $^1/_2$ c. brown rice flour
$^1/_2$ c. ground turkey (precooked)
2 eggs
$^1/_2$ c. dried cranberries
2 tbsp. honey
1 tsp. dried rosemary
1 tsp. ground cinnamon
CBD oil (see page 16 for dosage amounts)

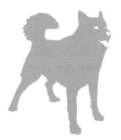

Preheat oven to 350°F. Peel and dice carrots. Place in a food processor and puree. Cook and mash sweet potatoes. Combine all ingredients together and mix until a dough forms. Roll out on a lightly floured surface to ¼" thickness. Use any shaped cookie cutter (or a knife) to cut into shapes. Line a cookie sheet with parchment paper (for easy cleanup), and place the cookies on the sheet (they can be rather close together, as they don't grow much while cooking).

Bake 25 to 30 minutes or until golden brown. Transfer and let cool completely on a wire rack. Store the cookies in an airtight container in the refrigerator. For more options, read the "Storage Tips" section on page 19.

CRANBERRIES

Cranberries are an antioxidant-rich superfruit. They are a good source of vitamin E, vitamin K, dietary fiber, vitamin C, and manganese. The polyphenols, antioxidants, and flavonoids in cranberries have been found to have beneficial qualities for kidney, bladder, and urinary tract health; dental health and gum disease; and cardiovascular health, as well as improvements in age-related declines of memory, balance, and coordination in animals.

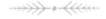

HOLIDAY HAPPINESS

For so many, the holiday season comes alive through baking. The kitchen becomes a place to create special cookies, breads, preserves—goodies that make friends and family feel special and welcomed, and that can be wrapped in festive papers to create the perfect gift. Absolutely no holiday celebration would be complete without the gingerbread man. Now your favorite four-legged family member gets their very own.

1 ½ c. oat flour
1 ½ c. brown rice flour
1 tsp. cinnamon
1 tsp. ground ginger
1 tsp. ground cloves
1 egg
¼ c. blackstrap molasses
¼ c. peanut butter (unsalted)
1 tbsp. apple cider vinegar
CBD oil (see page 16 for dosage amounts)
½ c. water (add slowly)

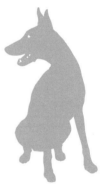

Preheat oven to 350°F. Combine all ingredients (except the water) together. Add water slowly and mix until a dough forms (if too dry, add more water; too wet, add a bit more flour). You may not need all the water if you reach a good consistency first. Roll out on a lightly floured surface to ¼" thickness. Use a gingerbread man cookie cutter (or any cookie cutter) to cut into shapes. Line a cookie sheet with parchment paper (for easy cleanup), and place the cookies on the sheet (they can be rather close together, as they don't grow much while cooking).

Bake 20 to 25 minutes or until golden brown. Transfer and let cool completely on a wire rack. Store the cookies in an airtight container in the refrigerator. For more options, read the "Storage Tips" section on page 19.

These are great treats to decorate and give out to all the dogs on your holiday lists (as long as their owners know that they contain CBD). There are some icing recipes on pages 171 and 173 that can be used with this recipe to make some truly special treats for your four-legged family members this holiday season.

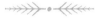

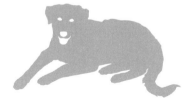

CHAPTER 2

DINER
DAYDREAM

The daily specials—all the classics

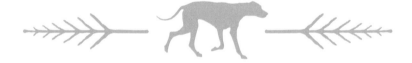

Don't you love going into one of those classic American diners and finding a sandwich menu that's several pages long and includes some one-of-a-kind concoctions? Now add the relaxing and healing properties of CBD to that, and imagine how your dog will feel when they get to sample from this menu. If you have several of these flavor varieties on hand, you can even let them choose their favorite for the day—just as you do at the diner!

Choose to use organic ingredients in these recipes, like we do!

SAGE CHICKEN

{ A SAVORY SNACK }

1 ½ c. oat flour
1 ½ c. brown rice flour
½ c. ground chicken (precooked)
½ c. oat bran
1 tsp. ground sage
1 egg
CBD oil (see page 16 for dosage amounts)
½ c. chicken broth (add slowly)

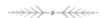

Preheat oven to 350°F. Combine all ingredients (except the broth) together. Add broth slowly and mix until a dough forms (if too dry, add more broth; too wet, add a bit more flour). You may not need all the broth if you reach a good consistency first. Roll out on a lightly floured surface to ¼" thickness. Use a cookie cutter (or a knife) to cut into shapes. Line a cookie sheet with parchment paper (for easy cleanup), and place the cookies on the sheet (they can be rather close together, as they don't grow much while cooking).

Bake 22 to 27 minutes or until golden brown. Transfer and let cool completely on a wire rack. Store the cookies in an airtight container in the refrigerator. For more options, read the "Storage Tips" section on page 19.

BROTH VS. GRAVY

Like the recipes in the cookbooks you use, the ones here feature ingredients that you would normally purchase from a store. One of these is chicken broth (or beef or vegetable broth). If you want to really spoil your dog (and the rest of your family), you can make these broths at home, then refrigerate them so you have them handy to use in your recipes. A broth is essentially the juice that's created when meat or vegetables are steamed or boiled. Don't substitute gravy, which is a broth-based food that's had other things mixed into it to thicken or stabilize it—usually cornstarch. Besides that, our recipes are corn free, as the grain is a potential source of allergies in dogs.

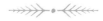

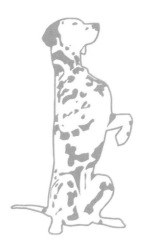

THE BARNYARD

{ A SIMPLE BACON, EGG & CHEESE }

1 ½ c. oat flour
1 ½ c. brown rice flour
½ c. shredded cheddar cheese
6 slices cooked bacon
2 eggs
CBD oil (see page 16 for dosage amounts)
¼ c. water (add slowly)

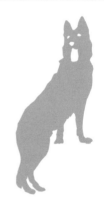

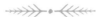

Preheat oven to 350°F. Combine all ingredients (except the water) together. Add water slowly and mix until a dough forms (if too dry, add more water; too wet, add a bit more flour). You may not need all the water if you reach a good consistency first. Roll out on a lightly floured surface to ¼" thickness. Use a cookie cutter (or a knife) to cut into shapes. Line a cookie sheet with parchment paper (for easy cleanup), and place the cookies on the sheet (they can be rather close together, as they don't grow much while cooking).

Bake 22 to 27 minutes or until golden brown. Transfer and let cool completely on a wire rack. Store the cookies in an airtight container in the refrigerator. For more options, read the "Storage Tips" section on page 19.

BACON IS NOT ALL THE SAME

Not all things are created equal, and this definitely applies to bacon. It is the favorite breakfast side, as well as quite arguably the most desirable piece of piggy there is. With that being said, we do recommend that you purchase natural bacon, which is not raised with any antibiotics and is free range and nitrite free. These characteristics make for a healthier treat, and it definitely is tastier too! While you're cooking it up for these treats, give it a taste. We are sure you'll notice the difference!

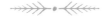

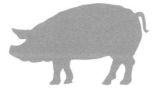

BEEF & CHEESE BOMB

{ IT'S JUST A PLAIN OLD CHEESEBURGER—
OH, SO TASTY }

1 ½ c. oat flour

1 ½ c. brown rice flour

1 egg

½ c. lean ground beef (precooked and drained)

½ c. shredded low-fat cheddar cheese

¼ c. tomato paste

CBD oil (see page 16 for dosage amounts)

½ c. water (add slowly)

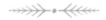

Preheat oven to 350°F. Combine all ingredients (except the water) together. Add water slowly and mix until a dough forms (if too dry, add more water; too wet, add a bit more flour). You may not need all the water if you reach a good consistency first. Roll out on a lightly floured surface to ¼" thickness. Use a round cookie cutter or the rim of an upside-down glass to cut into 2" circles. Line a cookie sheet with parchment paper (for easy cleanup), and place the cookies on the sheet (they can be rather close together, as they don't grow much while cooking).

Bake 22 to 27 minutes or until golden brown. Transfer and let cool completely on a wire rack. Store the cookies in an airtight container in the refrigerator. For more options, read the "Storage Tips" section on page 19.

PREPARING THE BEEF

We ask that you precook the ground beef in this and other recipes in this book because it results in the safest end product for your dog. Even if you start with organic, grass-fed beef (or other meat), you want to make sure that any harmful bacteria are cooked out and that you are draining as much of the fat off the cooked meat as possible before adding it to the other ingredients in these recipes.

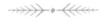

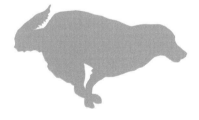

THE CHEESE GOBBLER

{ ...HOLD THE MAYO! }

1 ½ c. oat flour
1 ½ c. brown rice flour
½ c. grated Swiss cheese
½ c. ground turkey (precooked and drained)
½ c. oat bran
1 tbsp. dried parsley
1 egg
CBD oil (see page 16 for dosage amounts)
½ c. water (add slowly)

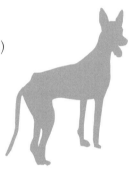

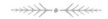

Preheat oven to 350°F. Combine all ingredients (except the water) together. Add water slowly and mix until a dough forms (if too dry, add more water; too wet, add a bit more flour). You may not need all the water if you reach a good consistency first. Roll out on a lightly floured surface to ¼" thickness. Use a cookie cutter (or a knife) to cut into shapes. Line a cookie sheet with parchment paper (for easy cleanup), and place the cookies on the sheet (they can be rather close together, as they don't grow much while cooking).

Bake 22 to 27 minutes or until golden brown. Transfer and let cool completely on a wire rack. Store the cookies in an airtight container in the refrigerator. For more options, read the "Storage Tips" section on page 19.

SUBSTITUTIONS: JUST DO IT!

The great thing about baking your own dog treats is that you can substitute many of the ingredients for items you have on hand or that you know your dog prefers. Since these flours are a little tricky to work with, I would avoid swapping those out, as the recipe will require a good amount of adjusting with a different flour. But the main "flavor" ingredients can easily be switched around. For example, this recipe calls for turkey and Swiss cheese. What if you have roast beef and provolone? Go ahead and use them instead. It's that easy throughout. If you want to swap tuna for salmon or chicken for turkey in a recipe, feel free. *Take note,* however: NEVER substitute an ingredient that may be toxic to dogs, such as onions, chocolate, raisins, macadamia nuts, or grapes.

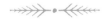

SWEET DREAMS ARE MADE OF CHEESE

{ LOVED BY KIDS & DOGS ALIKE }

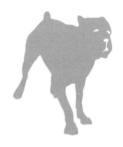

1 ½ c. oat flour
1 ½ c. brown rice flour
1 c. shredded low-fat cheddar cheese
½ c. grated Parmesan cheese
1 egg
CBD oil (see page 16 for dosage amounts)
½ c. water (add slowly)

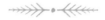

Preheat oven to 350°F. Combine all ingredients (except the water) together. Add water slowly and mix until a dough forms (if too dry, add more water; too wet, add a bit more flour). You may not need all the water if you reach a good consistency first. Roll out on a lightly floured surface to ¼" thickness. Use a cookie cutter (or a knife) to cut into shapes. Line a cookie sheet with parchment paper (for easy cleanup), and place the cookies on the sheet (they can be rather close together, as they don't grow much while cooking).

Bake 22 to 27 minutes or until golden brown. Transfer and let cool completely on a wire rack. Store the cookies in an airtight container in the refrigerator. For more options, read the "Storage Tips" section on page 19.

CHEESE IS ALWAYS A WINNER

OK, so let's cut to the chase: dogs love cheese. It's a plain and simple fact; that's why so many people use a slice of cheese to conceal their dog's medicine in (when necessary). We use cheese in a lot of our recipes for this very reason. You can always exchange cheeses too with one you have on hand.

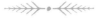

PIZZA MIND

{ NO CRUSTS HERE; THIS ONE'S ALL THEIRS }

FOR THE DOUGH:

1 ½ c. oat flour

1 ½ c. brown rice flour

1 egg

¼ c. low-fat ricotta cheese

CBD oil (see page 16 for dosage amounts)

⅓ c. water (add slowly)

FOR THE TOPPING:

6-oz. can tomato paste

1 c. shredded low-fat mozzarella cheese

1 tsp. dried basil

1 tsp. dried oregano

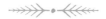

Preheat oven to 350°F. Combine all ingredients (except the water) together. Add water slowly and mix until a dough forms (if too dry, add more water; too wet, add a bit more flour). You may not need all the water if you reach a good consistency first. Roll out on a lightly floured surface to ¼" thickness. Use a round cookie cutter or the rim of an upside-down glass to cut 2" round circles out of the dough. Line a cookie sheet with parchment paper (for easy cleanup), and place the cookies on the sheet (they can be rather close together, as they don't grow much while cooking).

Now for the toppings. Spread the tomato paste on each first, then sprinkle the cheese and spices on top of each.

Bake 25 to 30 minutes or until golden brown. Transfer and let cool completely on a wire rack. Store the cookies in an airtight container in the refrigerator. For more options, read the "Storage Tips" section on page 19.

Alternates: For an extra twist, add a few slices of turkey, low-fat pepperoni, or diced grilled chicken on top of the pizzas before baking. Think of all those savory pizza toppings you love so much, or use some of your dog's favorite meats on top for an extra-special treat.

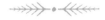

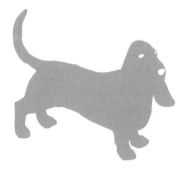

ARROZ CON POLLO

{ ¡MUY BUENO! }

1 ½ c. oat flour

1 ½ c. brown rice flour

½ c. ground chicken (precooked)

½ c. cooked brown rice

1 tbsp. dried parsley

1 tbsp. paprika

1 egg

CBD oil (see page 16 for dosage amounts)

½ c. water (or chicken broth—add slowly)

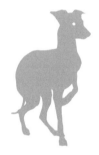

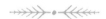

Preheat oven to 350°F. Combine all ingredients (except the water) together. Add water slowly and mix until a dough forms (if too dry, add more water; too wet, add a bit more flour). You may not need all the water if you reach a good consistency first. Roll out on a lightly floured surface to ¼" thickness. Use a cookie cutter (or a knife) to cut into shapes. Line a cookie sheet with parchment paper (for easy cleanup), and place the cookies on the sheet (they can be rather close together, as they don't grow much while cooking).

Bake 22 to 27 minutes or until golden brown. Transfer and let cool completely on a wire rack. Store the cookies in an airtight container in the refrigerator. For more options, read the "Storage Tips" section on page 19.

FOR THE SCHOLARLY DOG

Before they just gobble up these yummy treats, you may want to educate and inspire your dog by telling them what these Spanish words mean in English. It's so simple, it only takes a second. *Arroz* means rice, and pollo means chicken. Arroz con pollo is rice with chicken, or more familiarly, chicken and rice. Lesson learned.

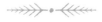

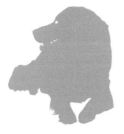

CHEESYGOING FRIES

{ THE LATE-NIGHT CLASSIC }

1 ½ c. oat flour
1 ½ c. brown rice flour
1 tsp. baking soda
2 tsp. baking powder
1 c. shredded low-fat cheddar cheese
1 egg
¼ c. extra-virgin olive oil
CBD oil (see page 16 for dosage amounts)
½ c. water (add slowly)

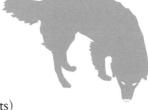

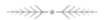

Preheat oven to 350°F. Combine all ingredients (except the water) together, reserving ½ c. cheddar cheese for the topping. Add water slowly and mix until a dough forms (if too dry, add more water; too wet, add a bit more flour). You may not need all the water if you reach a good consistency first. Roll the dough out on a lightly floured surface. Separate pieces and form sticks (about 3" long and ½" in diameter). Line a cookie sheet with parchment paper (for easy cleanup), and place the fries on the sheet (they can be rather close together, as they don't grow much while cooking). Sprinkle the remaining cheddar cheese on top of the fries.

Bake 22 to 27 minutes or until golden brown. Transfer and let cool completely on a wire rack. Store the fries in an airtight container in the refrigerator. For more options, read the "Storage Tips" section on page 19.

OILS

There are many kinds of oils available to cook with, and you may be tempted to use something other than extra-virgin olive oil. We list that kind of oil as an ingredient, however, because we feel that it is the kind that is best used by your dog's body. Most vegetable oils are soybean or corn based, and we prefer to use extra-virgin olive oil.

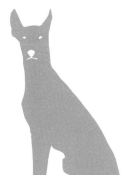

LIVER THE GOOD LIFE

{ GRANDPA'S FAVORITE—BUT NO ONIONS }

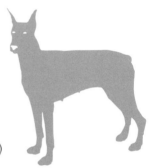

½ lb. raw beef or chicken livers
6 slices cooked bacon
1 ½ c. oat flour
1 ½ c. brown rice flour
1 c. oat bran
1 egg
CBD oil (see page 16 for dosage amounts)
½ c. water (add slowly)

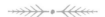

Preheat oven to 350°F. Puree livers in a food processor. Grind bacon into fine pieces in a food processor. Immediately clean the food processor afterward; you definitely don't want either of these pulverized meats drying in your appliance. Cleaning this up if they do is not easy.

Combine all ingredients (except the water) together. Add water slowly and mix until a dough forms (if too dry, add more water; too wet, add a bit more flour). You may not need all the water if you reach a good consistency first. Roll out on a lightly floured surface to ¼" thickness. Use a cookie cutter (or a knife) to cut into shapes. Line a cookie sheet with parchment paper (for easy cleanup), and place the cookies on the sheet (they can be rather close together, as they don't grow much while cooking).

Bake 25 to 30 minutes or until golden brown. Transfer and let cool completely on a wire rack. Store the cookies in an airtight container in the refrigerator. For more options, read the "Storage Tips" section on page 19.

Note: For crispier treats, do not take them out of the oven to cool. Turn the oven off and let them sit in there overnight. Store in the refrigerator once removed.

ONIONS—DEFINITELY A NO-NO

It has recently been reported that onions can be toxic (poisonous) to dogs (and cats). These foods have been shown to cause a form of hemolytic anemia in some animals who ingest them. Hemolytic anemia is a disease of the red blood cells. For this reason, we advise you not to use them in any of our recipes, or in any foods you prepare or give to your dog.

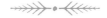

TREATS THAT FIT THE BILL

{ A SAVORY DUCK TREAT }

1 ½ c. oat flour

1 ½ c. brown rice flour

½ c. oat bran

½ c. ground duck breast (precooked and drained)

1 tsp. rosemary

1 egg

CBD oil (see page 16 for dosage amounts)

½ c. water (add slowly)

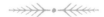

Preheat oven to 350°F. Combine all ingredients (except the water) together. Add water slowly and mix until a dough forms (if too dry, add more water; too wet, add a bit more flour). You may not need all the water if you reach a good consistency first. Roll out on a lightly floured surface to ¼" thickness. Use a cookie cutter (or a knife) to cut into shapes. Line a cookie sheet with parchment paper (for easy cleanup), and place the cookies on the sheet (they can be rather close together, as they don't grow much while cooking).

Bake 22 to 27 minutes or until golden brown. Transfer and let cool completely on a wire rack. Store the cookies in an airtight container in the refrigerator. For more options, read the "Storage Tips" section on page 19.

GAME BIRDS INSTEAD?

A lot of dogs these days are accustomed to eating some pretty delectable birds, including pheasant, duck, goose, quail, etc. If you happen to hunt or know a hunter and have easy access to these other delicious game birds, feel free to substitute any one of these meats for the duck. These are all great protein sources, as well as being less common, therefore making it less likely that there would be any built-in allergies to them.

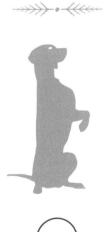

FINTASTIC SNACKS

{ FISH & CHIPS, THE IRISH SETTER OF SNACK FOODS }

1/2 c. cod (or another white fish)
1 1/2 c. oat flour
1 c. potato flour
1/2 c. oat bran
1 tsp. dill
1 egg
CBD oil (see page 16 for dosage amounts)
1/2 c. water (add slowly)

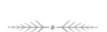

Preheat oven to 350°F. Cook the cod thoroughly (use as little oil as possible). Finely grind it in a food processor.

Combine all ingredients (except the water) together. Add water slowly and mix until a dough forms (if too dry, add more water; too wet, add a bit more flour). You may not need all the water if you reach a good consistency first. Roll out on a lightly floured surface to 1/4" thickness. Use a cookie cutter (or a knife) to cut into shapes. Line a cookie sheet with parchment paper (for easy cleanup), and place the cookies on the sheet (they can be rather close together, as they don't grow much while cooking).

Bake 22 to 27 minutes or until golden brown. Transfer and let cool completely on a wire rack. Store the cookies in an airtight container in the refrigerator. For more options, read the "Storage Tips" section on page 19.

FISH FOR DOGS!

It's pretty common knowledge that fish is good for both humans and dogs—but why? And what about contaminants like mercury or other toxins? To answer the first question, fish is a rich source of important omega-3 fatty acids. These are the ones that support the optimal functioning of the heart, eyes, immune system, skeletal system, and skin and coat. Supplementing with omega-3-rich foods can benefit such conditions as allergies, arthritis, heart disease, and even cancer. Of course, it's important to find high-quality sources of fish so that its benefits aren't outweighed by what may be contaminating it— including mercury. That is why we recommend using wild-caught fish in our recipes.

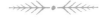

PUPPY POTSTICKERS

{ SOMETHING SPECIAL IN EVERY BITE! }

FOR THE DOUGH:

1 ½ c. oat flour

1 ½ c. brown rice flour

1 tsp. baking powder

1 egg

CBD oil (see page 16 for dosage amounts)

½ c. chicken broth (add slowly)

FILLING SUGGESTIONS:

Canned pumpkin

Cheese cubes (cheddar's always a favorite)

Small peeled apple pieces

Beef (precooked and ground or in small pieces)

Turkey (precooked and ground or in small pieces)

Bacon (precooked and crumbled)

Tuna

Peanut butter (unsalted)

Preheat oven to 350°F. Combine all dough ingredients (except the broth) together. Add broth slowly and mix until a dough forms (if too dry, add more broth; too wet, add a bit more flour). You may not need all the broth if you reach a good consistency first. Roll out on a lightly floured surface to ¼" thickness. Use a round cookie cutter or the rim of an upside-down glass to cut 2 ½" circles.

Place a small amount of any of the suggested fillings—or another of your dog's favorite things—in the center and press the edges up and together, making a little bundle. Line a cookie sheet with parchment paper (for easy cleanup), and place the cookies on the sheet (they can be rather close together, as they don't grow much while cooking).

Bake 25 to 30 minutes or until golden brown. Transfer and let cool completely on a wire rack. Store the cookies in an airtight container in the refrigerator. For more options, read the "Storage Tips" section on page 19.

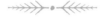

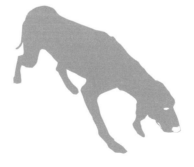

CHEESE ALL THAT

{ & A SIDE OF BACON }

6 slices cooked bacon
1 ½ c. oat flour
1 ½ c. brown rice flour
½ c. shredded low-fat cheddar cheese
1 egg
CBD oil (see page 16 for dosage amounts)
½ c. water (add slowly)

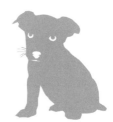

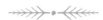

Preheat oven to 350°F. Cook bacon slices, then finely grind them in a food processor.

Combine all ingredients (except the water) together. Add water slowly and mix until a dough forms (if too dry, add more water; too wet, add a bit more flour). You may not need all the water if you reach a good consistency first.

Roll out on a lightly floured surface to ¼" thickness. Use a cookie cutter (or a knife) to cut into shapes. Line a cookie sheet with parchment paper (for easy cleanup), and place the cookies on the sheet (they can be rather close together, as they don't grow much while cooking).

Bake 22 to 27 minutes or until golden brown. Transfer and let cool completely on a wire rack. Store the cookies in an airtight container in the refrigerator. For more options, read the "Storage Tips" section on page 19.

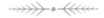

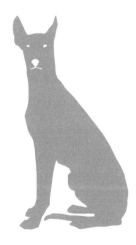

BEEF & TATERS

{ THE FUNDAMENTALS }

1 ½ c. oat flour
1 ½ c. potato flour
½ c. oat bran
½ c. lean ground beef (precooked and drained)
1 tsp. parsley
1 tsp. oregano
1 tsp. basil
1 egg
CBD oil (see page 16 for dosage amounts)
½ c. water (add slowly)

Preheat oven to 350°F. Combine all ingredients (except the water) together. Add water slowly and mix until a dough forms (if too dry, add more water; too wet, add a bit more flour). You may not need all the water if you reach a good consistency first.

Roll out on a lightly floured surface to ¼" thickness. Use a cookie cutter (or a knife) to cut into shapes. Line a cookie sheet with parchment paper (for easy cleanup), and place the cookies on the sheet (they can be rather close together, as they don't grow much while cooking).

Bake 22 to 27 minutes or until golden brown. Transfer and let cool completely on a wire rack. Store the cookies in an airtight container in the refrigerator. For more options, read the "Storage Tips" section on page 19.

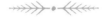

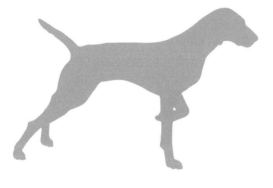

NOTHING CHEDDAR THAN THIS

{ GRANDMA'S FAVORITE }

1 c. raw chicken liver (or beef liver)

1 ½ c. oat flour

1 ½ c. brown rice flour

½ c. shredded low-fat cheddar cheese

1 egg

CBD oil (see page 16 for dosage amounts)

½ c. water (add slowly)

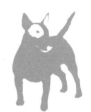

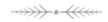

Preheat oven to 350°F. Puree the liver in a food processor. Immediately clean the food processor afterward; once the liver dries it is very hard and unpleasant to get out of there.

Combine all ingredients (except the water) together. Add water slowly and mix until a dough forms (if too dry, add more water; too wet, add a bit more flour). You may not need all the water if you reach a good consistency first. Roll out on a lightly floured surface to ¼" thickness. Use a cookie cutter (or a knife) to cut into shapes. Line a cookie sheet with parchment paper (for easy cleanup), and place the cookies on the sheet (they can be rather close together, as they don't grow much while cooking).

Bake 22 to 27 minutes or until golden brown. Transfer and let cool completely on a wire rack. Store the cookies in an airtight container in the refrigerator. For more options, read the "Storage Tips" section on page 19.

LIVER—IT'S TIME TO LOVE IT

Liver is an organ meat, and while all carnivores have been feasting on and benefiting from organ meats for as long as they've (we've) been roaming the planet, in the United States today, liver is much maligned as smelly and slimy. Add to that a reputation for being high in cholesterol, and it's no surprise that it's not a popular choice for the family dinner table. But liver has long been an acceptable and desired ingredient in dog food and treats—and it's no wonder. Liver is loaded with vitamin A (retinol), which is good for your eyes, skin, and mucous membranes. It also contains vitamins E, D, and K, is packed with essential minerals, is a high-quality protein source, and is rich in omega-3 and omega-6 fatty acids. All these are great for your dog—and for you! One additional note: because the liver is the detoxifying organ in the body, purchase meat that is as limited in its exposure to toxin processing as possible, such as an organic cut.

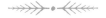

PECANS & MOLASSES & OATS

{ OH MY! }

1 ½ c. oat flour

1 ½ c. brown rice flour

¼ c. finely ground pecans

½ c. rolled oats (the old-fashioned kind, not instant)

¼ c. blackstrap molasses

1 egg

CBD oil (see page 16 for dosage amounts)

½ c. water (add slowly)

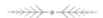

Preheat oven to 350°F. Combine all ingredients (except the water) together. Add water slowly and mix until a dough forms (if too dry, add more water; too wet, add a bit more flour). You may not need all the water if you reach a good consistency first. Roll out on a lightly floured surface to ¼" thickness. Use a cookie cutter (or a knife) to cut into shapes. Line a cookie sheet with parchment paper (for easy cleanup), and place the cookies on the sheet (they can be rather close together, as they don't grow much while cooking).

Bake 22 to 27 minutes or until golden brown. Transfer and let cool completely on a wire rack. Store the cookies in an airtight container in the refrigerator. For more options, read the "Storage Tips" section on page 19.

BENEFITS OF MOLASSES

If you're looking for alternative sources of sweeteners in a wide range of foods, one that you should consider is blackstrap molasses. This thick syrup is the by-product of refining sugar: it is the third boiling of the sugar syrup, so it is technically the concentrate left over after the sugar's sucrose has been crystallized. What's left are lots of beneficial minerals—iron, copper, manganese, magnesium, potassium, and calcium—as well as a dose of vitamin B_6. While the taste of blackstrap molasses takes some getting used to (though baked beans or ginger snaps wouldn't be the same without it), dogs are typically less discriminating. Ours love the flavor, and we're sure yours will too.

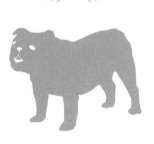

SOUP-ER BISCUITS

{ BEEF BARLEY IN BISCUIT FORM }

½ c. pureed carrots
½ c. pureed celery
2 c. oat flour
1 ½ c. barley flour
½ c. lean ground beef (precooked and drained)
½ c. oat bran
1 tsp. parsley
1 tsp. dill
1 egg
CBD oil (see page 16 for dosage amounts)
½ c. water (add slowly)

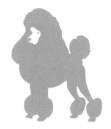

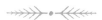

Preheat oven to 350°F. Peel and dice carrots and celery, then puree in a food processor.

Combine all ingredients (except the water) together. Add water slowly and mix until a dough forms (if too dry, add more water; too wet, add a bit more flour). You may not need all the water if you reach a good consistency first. Roll out on a lightly floured surface to ¼" thickness. Use a cookie cutter (or a knife) to cut into shapes. Line a cookie sheet with parchment paper (for easy cleanup), and place the cookies on the sheet (they can be rather close together, as they don't grow much while cooking).

Bake 22 to 27 minutes or until golden brown. Transfer and let cool completely on a wire rack. Store the cookies in an airtight container in the refrigerator. For more options, read the "Storage Tips" section on page 19.

BENEFITS OF BARLEY

Like wheat, barley is a grain that produces seeds that are then ground to produce flour. There are several benefits of barley compared to wheat: barley is higher in fiber, contains vitamin E, and has more thiamin, riboflavin, lysine, and essential fatty acids.

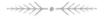

SUSHI ROLL

{ MAKE THIS SALMON FAVORITE AN EASY TREAT }

1 1/2 c. oat flour
1 1/2 c. brown rice flour
6-oz. can wild-caught salmon
1/2 c. oat bran
1 tsp. dill
1/2 c. low-fat cream cheese
1 egg
CBD oil (see page 16 for dosage amounts)
1/2 c. water (add slowly)

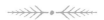

Preheat oven to 350°F. Combine all ingredients (except the water) together. Add water slowly and mix until a dough forms (if too dry, add more water; too wet, add a bit more flour). You may not need all the water if you reach a good consistency first. Roll out on a lightly floured surface to 1/4" thickness. Use a cookie cutter (or a knife) to cut into shapes. Line a cookie sheet with parchment paper (for easy cleanup), and place the cookies on the sheet (they can be rather close together, as they don't grow much while cooking).

Bake 22 to 27 minutes or until golden brown. Transfer and let cool completely on a wire rack. Store the cookies in an airtight container in the refrigerator. For more options, read the "Storage Tips" section on page 19.

SALMON

Salmon is low in calories and saturated fat, while high in protein. It is a wonderful source of the amazingly beneficial omega-3 fatty acids, vitamin D, selenium, B vitamins, and magnesium, which are excellent for skin, coat, and heart health. And salmon is a great alternative protein source for dogs with allergies to the more common proteins of chicken and beef.

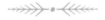

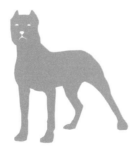

RELAXATION OPPOR-TUNA-TY

{ FRIES NOT INCLUDED }

6-oz. can albacore tuna (in water)
1 $\frac{1}{2}$ c. oat flour
1 $\frac{1}{2}$ c. brown rice flour
$\frac{1}{2}$ c. oat bran
$\frac{1}{2}$ c. shredded low-fat cheddar cheese
1 egg
CBD oil (see page 16 for dosage amounts)
$\frac{1}{4}$ c. water (add slowly)

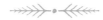

Preheat oven to 350°F. Pour entire contents of can of tuna (including all water and juices) into a food processor and finely grind.

Combine all ingredients (except the water) together. Add water slowly and mix until a dough forms (if too dry, add more water; too wet, add a bit more flour). You may not need all the water if you reach a good consistency first.

Roll out on a lightly floured surface to ¼" thickness. Use a cookie cutter (or a knife) to cut into shapes. Line a cookie sheet with parchment paper (for easy cleanup), and place the cookies on the sheet (they can be rather close together, as they don't grow much while cooking).

Bake 22 to 27 minutes or until golden brown. Transfer and let cool completely on a wire rack. Store the cookies in an airtight container in the refrigerator. For more options, read the "Storage Tips" section on page 19.

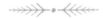

CHAPTER 3

UNWIND & DINE

For dogs who live in the lap of luxury

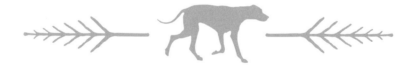

The recipes in Chapter 2 were created for that down-home kind of feeling: comfort food with a kick. These recipes—while equally delicious—are for the more adventurous palate, or to be served to your too-classy pooch on special occasions (and let's face it, every day with your dog is a special occasion!). For the aging and elegant, these refined recipes will help those aching joints. For the young and fabulous, these will help relax them so they can dine in style. Bon appétit!

Choose to use organic ingredients in these recipes, like we do!

ANTIPASTO
{ THE BEST IS ALWAYS THE CHEESY BREAD }

....

$^{1}/_{2}$ c. low-fat shredded mozzarella cheese (for topping)

1 $^{1}/_{2}$ c. oat flour

1 $^{1}/_{2}$ c. brown rice flour

1 tsp. baking soda

2 tsp. baking powder

1 tsp. dried rosemary

$^{1}/_{2}$ c. grated Parmesan cheese

1 egg

$^{1}/_{4}$ c. olive oil

CBD oil (see page 16 for dosage amounts)

$^{1}/_{2}$ c. water (add slowly)

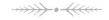

Preheat oven to 350°F. Set the mozzarella cheese aside to be used later as a topping. Combine all other ingredients (except the water) together. Add water slowly and mix until a dough forms (if too dry, add more water; too wet, add a bit more flour). You may not need all the water if you reach a good consistency first. Roll out on a lightly floured surface to $^{1}/_{4}$" thickness.

Use a cookie cutter (or a knife) to cut into shapes. Line a cookie sheet with parchment paper (for easy cleanup), and place the cookies on the sheet (they can be rather close together, as they don't grow much while cooking). Sprinkle the mozzarella cheese on top of the cookies.

Bake 20 to 25 minutes or until golden brown. Transfer and let cool completely on a wire rack. Store the cookies in an airtight container in the refrigerator. For more options, read the "Storage Tips" section on page 19.

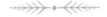

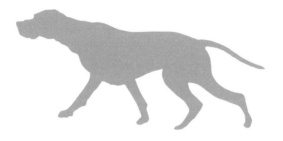

CHEESE LOUISE!

{ WHEN ONE CHEESE JUST ISN'T ENOUGH }

1 1/2 c. oat flour
1 1/2 c. brown rice flour
1/2 c. grated Parmesan cheese
1/2 c. low-fat ricotta cheese
1/2 c. shredded low-fat mozzarella
1/2 c. grated romano cheese
1 tsp. dried basil
1 tsp. dried oregano
1 egg
CBD oil (see page 16 for dosage amounts)
1/2 c. water (add slowly)

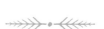

Preheat oven to 350°F. Combine all ingredients (except the water) together. Add water slowly and mix until a dough forms (if too dry, add more water; too wet, add a bit more flour). You may not need all the water if you reach a good consistency first. Roll out on a lightly floured surface to 1/4" thickness.

Use a cookie cutter (or a knife) to cut into shapes. Line a cookie sheet with parchment paper (for easy cleanup), and place the cookies on the sheet (they can be rather close together, as they don't grow much while cooking).

Bake 22 to 27 minutes or until golden brown. Transfer and let cool completely on a wire rack. Store the cookies in an airtight container in the refrigerator. For more options, read the "Storage Tips" section on page 19.

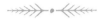

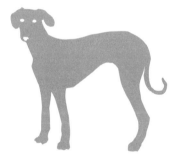

POULTRY IN MOTION

{ A SAVORY & DELISH TREAT FOR ANY DOG }

1 ½ c. oat flour
1 ½ c. brown rice flour
½ c. ground chicken (precooked)
1 tbsp. rosemary
1 tbsp. sage
1 tbsp. grated Parmesan cheese
1 egg
CBD oil (see page 16 for dosage amounts)
½ c. chicken broth (add slowly)

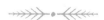

Preheat oven to 350°F. Combine all ingredients (except the broth) together. Add broth slowly and mix until a dough forms (if too dry, add more broth; too wet, add a bit more flour). You may not need all the broth if you reach a good consistency first. Roll out on a lightly floured surface to ¼" thickness.

Use a cookie cutter (or a knife) to cut into shapes. Line a cookie sheet with parchment paper (for easy cleanup), and place the cookies on the sheet (they can be rather close together, as they don't grow much while cooking).

Bake 22 to 27 minutes or until golden brown. Transfer and let cool completely on a wire rack. Store the cookies in an airtight container in the refrigerator. For more options, read the "Storage Tips" section on page 19.

LICKIN' THEIR CHOPS
FOR CHICKEN

Chicken is an ingredient in many dog foods, and for good reason. Besides being a protein that dogs enjoy, it is one of the best meat sources of protein. It packs a good dose of amino acids and is easily digestible. Like other meat sources, it's important to select the finest cuts from the best sources to optimize the nutritional benefits. With the good, there is also the bad. Unfortunately, more dogs are becoming allergic to chicken, as it is common in so many foods. If your dog is allergic to chicken, feel free to substitute turkey, duck, or any other protein in the recipes that call for chicken.

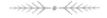

SIZZLING STEAK

{ A SOUTHWESTERN-STYLE TREAT FOR ALL }

1 ½ c. oat flour
1 ½ c. brown rice flour
½ c. lean ground beef (precooked and drained)
1 ½ c. tightly packed spinach leaves
1 tbsp. sesame seeds
¼ tsp. paprika
1 egg
CBD oil (see page 16 for dosage amounts)
½ c. water (add slowly)

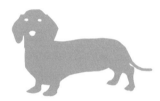

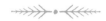

Preheat oven to 350°F. Combine all ingredients (except the water) together. Add water slowly and mix until a dough forms (if too dry, add more water; too wet, add a bit more flour). You may not need all the water if you reach a good consistency first. Roll out on a lightly floured surface to ¼" thickness. Use a cookie cutter (or a knife) to cut into shapes. Line a cookie sheet with parchment paper (for easy cleanup), and place the cookies on the sheet (they can be rather close together, as they don't grow much while cooking).

Bake 22 to 27 minutes or until golden brown. Transfer and let cool completely on a wire rack. Store the cookies in an airtight container in the refrigerator. For more options, read the "Storage Tips" section on page 19.

SUBSTITUTIONS ABOUND

Just a little reminder that we've already been over, but in case you missed it or forgot: substitutions! Feel free to swap out the beef for another protein. Maybe your dog doesn't digest beef all that well, just like a lot of people. Beef can be a bit tough to digest (leading to that all-too-well-known stinky butt). If that happens to your dog, then we recommend swapping out the beef for an alternative protein, such as venison or bison (which tend to be a lot better for those with beef sensitivities). Also, say you have kale in the fridge; you can use that instead of the spinach. Always keep in mind not to substitute with anything toxic to dogs, but there are a lot of options for quick and easy switches that you can do with what you have on hand.

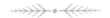

POTLUCK PASTRIES

{ A LITTLE BIT OF THIS, A LITTLE BIT OF THAT }

$\frac{1}{2}$ c. ground chicken (precooked)

$\frac{1}{2}$ c. ground pork (precooked)

6 slices cooked bacon

1 $\frac{1}{2}$ c. oat flour

1 $\frac{1}{2}$ c. brown rice flour

$\frac{1}{2}$ c. applesauce (unsweetened)

1 tsp. sage

$\frac{1}{2}$ c. grated Parmesan cheese

2 eggs

CBD oil (see page 16 for dosage amounts)

$\frac{1}{4}$ c. water (add slowly)

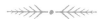

Preheat oven to 350°F. Finely grind the chicken, pork, and bacon in a food processor.

Combine all ingredients (except the water) together. Add water slowly and mix until a dough forms (if too dry, add more water; too wet, add a bit more flour). You may not need all the water if you reach a good consistency first. Roll out on a lightly floured surface to $\frac{1}{4}$" thickness. Use a cookie cutter (or a knife) to cut into shapes. Line a cookie sheet with parchment paper (for easy cleanup), and place the cookies on the sheet (they can be rather close together, as they don't grow much while cooking).

Bake 22 to 27 minutes or until golden brown. Transfer and let cool completely on a wire rack. Store the cookies in an airtight container in the refrigerator. For more options, read the "Storage Tips" section on page 19.

———>>>·<<<———

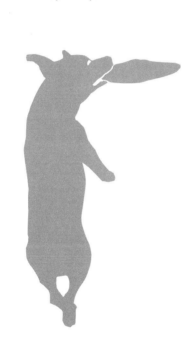

APPLE CHEDDAR BACON BISCUITS

{ REFINED & REFRESHING }

6 slices cooked bacon

1 ½ c. oat flour

1 ½ c. brown rice flour

½ c. shredded low-fat cheddar cheese

½ c. applesauce (unsweetened)

½ c. rolled oats (the old-fashioned kind, not instant)

1 egg

CBD oil (see page 16 for dosage amounts)

⅓ c. water (add slowly)

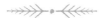

Preheat oven to 350°F. Finely grind the bacon in a food processor.

Combine all ingredients (except the water) together. Add water slowly and mix until a dough forms (if too dry, add more water; too wet, add a bit more flour). You may not need all the water if you reach a good consistency first.

Roll out on a lightly floured surface to ¼" thickness. Use a cookie cutter (or a knife) to cut into shapes. Line a cookie sheet with parchment paper (for easy cleanup), and place the cookies on the sheet (they can be rather close together, as they don't grow much while cooking).

Bake 22 to 27 minutes or until golden brown. Transfer and let cool completely on a wire rack. Store the cookies in an airtight container in the refrigerator. For more options, read the "Storage Tips" section on page 19.

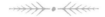

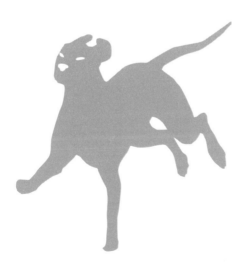

MAMMA MIA

{ HERE WE DOUGH AGAIN }

$\frac{1}{2}$ c. pureed roasted red peppers (optional)

1 $\frac{1}{2}$ c. oat flour

1 $\frac{1}{2}$ c. brown rice flour

6-oz. can tomato paste

$\frac{1}{2}$ c. fresh mozzarella, finely chopped

$\frac{1}{2}$ c. grated Parmesan cheese

1 tsp. dried rosemary

1 tsp. dried oregano

1 tsp. dried basil

1 egg

CBD oil (see page 16 for dosage amounts)

$\frac{1}{2}$ c. water (add slowly)

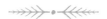

Preheat oven to 350°F. If using roasted red peppers, puree these in a food processor before doing anything else.

Combine all ingredients (except the water) together. Add water slowly and mix until a dough forms (if too dry, add more water; too wet, add a bit more flour). You may not need all the water if you reach a good consistency first. Roll out on a lightly floured surface to $\frac{1}{4}$" thickness. Use a cookie cutter (or a knife) to cut into shapes. Line a cookie sheet with parchment paper (for easy cleanup), and place the cookies on the sheet (they can be rather close together, as they don't grow much while cooking).

Bake 22 to 27 minutes or until golden brown. Transfer and let cool completely on a wire rack. Store the cookies in an airtight container in the refrigerator. For more options, read the "Storage Tips" section on page 19.

ROSEMARY—FOR MORE THAN JUST SEASONING

Rosemary—like sage and thyme—is traditionally used to season foods, particularly roasted meats and vegetables. It is becoming more and more appreciated for its medicinal as well as gustatory benefits. Rosemary is a natural antibiotic and antiseptic. It also increases blood flow to the brain, aids in memory, and, when inhaled, rejuvenates the senses. It is a potent herb, and a little goes a long way—we could all use a little more often, though.

PLENTY OF FISH IN THE CBD

{ A CATCHY TREAT }

6-oz. can wild-caught tuna
$1/2$ c. tightly packed arugula leaves
$1 1/2$ c. oat flour
$1 1/2$ c. brown rice flour
$1/2$ c. sesame seeds
$1/2$ c. finely ground peanuts
1 tbsp. honey
1 egg
CBD oil (see page 16 for dosage amounts)
$1/2$ c. water (add slowly)

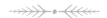

Preheat oven to 350°F. Empty entire contents of tuna can (including liquid and juices) into a food processor and puree it along with the arugula leaves.

Combine all ingredients (except the water) together. Add water slowly and mix until a dough forms (if too dry, add more water; too wet, add a bit more flour). You may not need all the water if you reach a good consistency first. Roll out on a lightly floured surface to $1/4"$ thickness. Use a cookie cutter (or a knife) to cut into shapes. Line a cookie sheet with parchment paper (for easy cleanup), and place the cookies on the sheet (they can be rather close together, as they don't grow much while cooking).

Bake 22 to 27 minutes or until golden brown. Transfer and let cool completely on a wire rack. Store the cookies in an airtight container in the refrigerator. For more options, read the "Storage Tips" section on page 19.

NUTS—LET'S EXPLORE

Many of the recipes in this book contain peanuts, because what dog doesn't love peanut butter? OK, we've heard of a few, but they are definitely in the minority. Other nuts that are good for dogs (and people) include cashews and almonds. Nuts are an excellent source of protein. But keep in mind that they are also high in fat. One nut to never feed your dog is the macadamia nut. While the exact source of its toxicity is still not known, it is associated with producing muscle tremors and partial paralysis in dogs. If you're going to get nutty, go for the good ones.

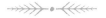

RE-FLAX WITH A SCONE

{ A LITTLE FLAXSEED TO ENHANCE
YOUR DOG'S NATURAL BEAUTY }

1 ½ c. oat flour

1 ½ c. brown rice flour

½ c. flaxseed meal (or flaxseeds)

½ c. ground peanuts (unsalted)

½ c. dried cranberries

3 tbsp. sesame seeds

1 egg

CBD oil (see page 16 for dosage amounts)

½ c. water (add slowly)

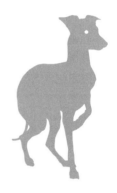

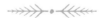

Preheat oven to 350°F. Combine all ingredients (except the water) together. Add water slowly and mix until a dough forms (if too dry, add more water; too wet, add a bit more flour). You may not need all the water if you reach a good consistency first. Roll out on a lightly floured surface to ¼" thickness. Use a cookie cutter (or a knife) to cut into shapes. Line a cookie sheet with parchment paper (for easy cleanup), and place the cookies on the sheet (they can be rather close together, as they don't grow much while cooking).

Bake 22 to 27 minutes or until golden brown. Transfer and let cool completely on a wire rack. Store the cookies in an airtight container in the refrigerator. For more options, read the "Storage Tips" section on page 19.

FLAXSEED

The seeds of the flax plant have been cultivated for human consumption for millennia. Flaxseed contains lignans, which are particularly beneficial to the female reproductive system. The fiber in flaxseed acts as a natural laxative to aid in digestion; in the intestine, it helps coat the lining, reducing the incidence of constipation, gastritis, and colon conditions. Using ground flaxseed in recipes certainly adds beneficial fiber and digestive support.

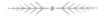

THE SO-FISH-TICATED
SPECIAL

{ THE UPTOWN WAY TO START THE DAY }

....

4 oz. lox
1 ½ c. oat flour
1 ½ c. brown rice flour
4 oz. low-fat cream cheese (at room temperature)
½ c. oat bran
1 tsp. dill
1 egg
CBD oil (see page 16 for dosage amounts)
½ c. water (add slowly)

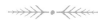

Preheat oven to 350°F. Slice lox and finely grind it in a food processor.

Combine all ingredients (except the water) together. Add water slowly and mix until a dough forms (if too dry, add more water; too wet, add a bit more flour). You may not need all the water if you reach a good consistency first. Roll out on a lightly floured surface to ¼" thickness. Use a cookie cutter (or a knife) to cut into shapes. Line a cookie sheet with parchment paper (for easy cleanup), and place the cookies on the sheet (they can be rather close together, as they don't grow much while cooking).

Bake 22 to 27 minutes or until golden brown. Transfer and let cool completely on a wire rack. Store the cookies in an airtight container in the refrigerator. For more options, read the "Storage Tips" section on page 19.

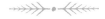

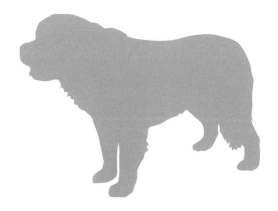

TART OF TARTS

{ DELECTABLE QUICHES FOR THAT
EXTRA-SPECIAL PUP }

....

¹/₂ c. pureed carrots
¹/₂ c. tightly packed spinach leaves
¹/₂ c. lean ground pork (precooked and drained)
1 ¹/₂ c. oat flour
¹/₂ c. oat bran
2 eggs
¹/₂ c. low-fat cottage cheese
1 tsp. basil
CBD oil (see page 16 for dosage amounts)

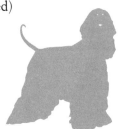

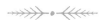

Preheat oven to 350°F. Peel, dice, and puree carrots in a food processor. Puree spinach leaves in a food processor until smooth. Grind the drained pork in a food processor.

Combine all ingredients together and mix thoroughly. Spray cooking spray thoroughly into a mini muffin pan (or a regular muffin pan). Push the mixture evenly into the pan (the consistency will be similar to meatloaf), coming close to the top (the mix will not rise very much).

Bake 20 to 25 minutes if using the mini muffin pan or 30 to 35 minutes if using a regular-sized muffin pan. Quiches are done when a toothpick inserted into the center comes out clean. Remove from the oven and let cool completely on a wire rack. Store in an airtight container in the refrigerator. For more options, read the "Storage Tips" section on page 19.

Note: A dollop of nonfat cream cheese or sour cream on top of these makes them an even more special treat. These are also a great option to vary the ingredients to make different-flavored quiches based on your dog's favorite things. Here are a few suggesstions:

- Swap the pork for beef and the cottage cheese for Swiss cheese

- Swap the pork for bacon and the cottage cheese for cheddar cheese

- Swap the pork for turkey and the cottage cheese for Swiss cheese

The possibilities are endless....

SPINACH—LEAN & GREEN

There must be something in spinach that enables Popeye to "fight to the finish" after he eats it. That "something" is a solid helping of fiber, the minerals calcium and potassium, and the vitamins A, B_6, and K. Spinach also has twice the iron content of most other greens, and it is a recognized source of antioxidants. Avoid Popeye's source—canned spinach—and instead choose organically grown regular or baby spinach and serve it lightly steamed or raw (chopped up finely).

AMBROSIA

{ A TREAT WORTHY OF GREEK GODS }

1 c. tightly packed spinach leaves
1 ½ c. oat flour
1 ½ c. brown rice flour
½ c. feta cheese
1 egg
CBD oil (see page 16 for dosage amounts)
½ c. water (add slowly)

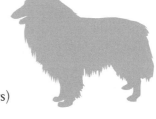

Preheat oven to 350°F. Puree spinach in a food processor.

Combine all ingredients (except the water) together. Add water slowly and mix until a dough forms (if too dry, add more water; too wet, add a bit more flour). You may not need all the water if you reach a good consistency first. Roll out on a lightly floured surface to ¼" thickness. Use a cookie cutter (or a knife) to cut into shapes. Line a cookie sheet with parchment paper (for easy cleanup), and place the cookies on the sheet (they can be rather close together, as they don't grow much while cooking).

Bake 25 to 30 minutes or until golden brown. Transfer and let cool completely on a wire rack. Store the cookies in an airtight container in the refrigerator. For more options, read the "Storage Tips" section on page 19.

PUPPY PÂTÉ

{ LIVER FOR YOUR LOVED ONES }

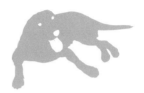

½ c. raw chicken (or beef) livers

2 c. oat flour

½ c. oat bran

2 eggs

CBD oil (see page 16 for dosage amounts)

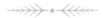

Preheat oven to 350°F. Puree the livers in a food processor. Immediately clean out the food processor afterward. Liver is very hard to get out once it dries, trust us.

Combine all ingredients together and mix thoroughly. Line a 9" square pan with parchment paper (you'll thank us for this) and pour the mixture in.

Bake 40 to 45 minutes or until the sides seem to be loosening from the pan. Cut into bite-sized pieces and let cool completely in the pan. Store the cookies in an airtight container in the refrigerator. For more options, read the "Storage Tips" section on page 19.

QUIRKY TURKEY

{ A THANKSGIVING FEAST IN A COOKIE }

$\frac{1}{2}$ c. ground turkey (precooked and drained)

1 $\frac{1}{2}$ c. oat flour

1 $\frac{1}{2}$ c. brown rice flour

$\frac{1}{2}$ c. oat bran

$\frac{1}{2}$ c. sweet potato or yams (precooked and mashed, or canned)

1 tsp. parsley

1 tsp. sage

1 tsp. rosemary

$\frac{1}{2}$ c. dried cranberries

1 egg

CBD oil (see page 16 for dosage amounts)

$\frac{1}{2}$ c. water (add slowly)

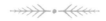

Preheat oven to 350°F. Grind the turkey in a food processor.

Combine all ingredients (except the water) together. Add water slowly and mix until a dough forms (if too dry, add more water; too wet, add a bit more flour). You may not need all the water if you reach a good consistency first. Roll the dough into 1" balls and place on a cookie sheet lined with parchment paper (for easier cleanup). Treats can be placed close together, as they don't spread while cooking.

Bake for 25 to 30 minutes or until golden brown. Transfer and let cool completely on a wire rack. Store the cookies in an airtight container in the refrigerator. For more options, read the "Storage Tips" section on page 19.

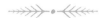

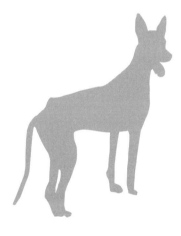

LET'S GET THE MEATBALL ROLLING

{ ALL IT NEEDS IS A LITTLE MARINARA }

2 lbs. raw, lean ground beef (or turkey)

½ c. grated Parmesan cheese

½ c. oat bran

1 tsp. dried oregano

1 tsp. dried parsley

1 tsp. dried basil

1 egg

CBD oil (see page 16 for dosage amounts)

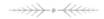

Preheat oven to 350°F. Combine all ingredients together and mix thoroughly. Roll the mixture into 1" balls and place on a cookie sheet lined with parchment paper (makes for easier cleanup). We recommend using rubber or latex gloves to form and roll the meatballs. It's a lot more pleasant that way.

Bake 15 to 20 minutes or until evenly browned and cooked through. Remove from the oven and let cool. Store in an airtight container in the refrigerator. For more options, read the "Storage Tips" section on page 19.

Notes: These freeze very well. We recommend placing a small amount in the refrigerator and the rest in a bag in the freezer. When you need more, you have them ready and on hand.

This is a great item to alternate proteins in. You can do 1 lb. beef with 1 lb. pork to make a mixed meatball. You can also use chicken or turkey to make a poultry version of this recipe.

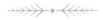

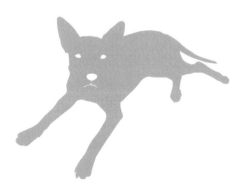

CHICKEN & BROCCOLI

{ STIR-FRY IN A BISCUIT }

1 ½ c. oat flour

1 ½ c. brown rice flour

½ c. oat bran

½ c. ground chicken (precooked)

½ c. pureed broccoli

2 tbsp. blackstrap molasses

1 egg

CBD oil (see page 16 for dosage amounts)

½ c. water (add slowly)

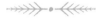

Preheat oven to 350°F. Drain the chicken, then grind in a food processor.

Combine all ingredients (except the water) together. Add water slowly and mix until a dough forms (if too dry, add more water; too wet, add a bit more flour). You may not need all the water if you reach a good consistency first. Roll out on a lightly floured surface to ¼" thickness. Use a cookie cutter (or a knife) to cut into shapes. Line a cookie sheet with parchment paper (for easy cleanup), and place the cookies on the sheet (they can be rather close together, as they don't grow much while cooking).

Bake 22 to 27 minutes or until golden brown. Transfer and let cool completely on a wire rack. Store the cookies in an airtight container in the refrigerator. For more options, read the "Storage Tips" section on page 19.

BROCCOLI—IT'S HARD TO BEAT

If you're looking for a veggie that packs a wallop of cancer-fighting phytochemicals as well as a solid dose of vitamin C, beta-carotene, folic acid, and calcium, then look no farther than the fresh, organic broccoli at your grocery store or farmers market. Chop or puree it raw before adding it to your dog's meals (or treats), or lightly steam it and cut it up—using the broth created by the steam too. Good stuff!

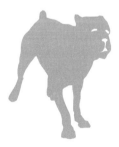

CHAPTER 4

SWEET
SERENITY

A little something for the sweet tooth

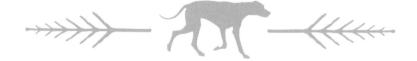

At the end of a long, stressful day, sometimes all you want to do is sit down and enjoy a sweet treat. With these recipes, you can give your best friends the opportunity to de-stress just like you do. Here are some treats that won't upset their digestive system and that aren't harmful (remember, never give chocolate to dogs!). With this wide selection of recipes to choose from, you have lots of options to charm and chillax your companions. Reward your sweet pups with some sweets!

Choose to use organic ingredients in these recipes, like we do!

THE ORIGINAL

{ THE KEYSTONE TO ANY COOKIE JAR– THE DOG-SAFE VERSION OF THE CHOCOLATE CHIP COOKIE }

1 ½ c. oat flour

1 ½ c. brown rice flour

½ c. carob chips (do NOT substitute with chocolate)

1 egg

1 tsp. vanilla

CBD oil (see page 16 for dosage amounts)

½ c. water (add slowly)

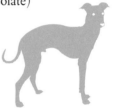

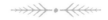

Preheat oven to 350°F. Combine all ingredients (except the water) together. Add water slowly and mix until a dough forms (if too dry, add more water; too wet, add a bit more flour). You may not need all the water if you reach a good consistency first. Roll into small balls (about 1" in diameter) and place on an ungreased cookie sheet (they can be rather close together, as they don't spread while cooking). Press each one down with your hand to flatten the cookies.

Bake 22 to 27 minutes or until golden brown. Transfer and let cool completely on a wire rack. Store the cookies in an airtight container in the refrigerator. For more options, read the "Storage Tips" section on page 19.

CAROB

Carob pods come from carob trees, which are small evergreen shrubs native to the Mediterranean. Before the use of sugar cane, carob was used as a natural sweetener. In fact, the pods have a taste reminiscent of sweetened cocoa, but without the theobromine, caffeine, or other psychoactive properties of cocoa (which are potentially lethal for dogs). Mixed with saturated fats, carob bars and chips can be safely substituted for chocolate. It is important to remember never to give a dog chocolate.

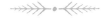

CINNAMON HONEY COOKIES

{ NOW DOGS HAVE THEIR OWN SNICKERDOODLES }

1 ½ c. oat flour
1 ½ c. brown rice flour
2 tsp. cinnamon
1 egg
¼ c. honey
1 tsp. vanilla
CBD oil (see page 16 for dosage amounts)
½ c. water (add slowly)

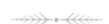

Preheat oven to 350°F. Combine all ingredients (except the water) together. Add water slowly and mix until a dough forms (if too dry, add more water; too wet, add a bit more flour). You may not need all the water if you reach a good consistency first. Spoon out the mixture and roll into balls (about 1" in diameter). Line a cookie sheet with parchment paper (for easy cleanup), and place the cookies on the sheet (they can be rather close together, as they don't grow much while cooking). Using a fork, press down the balls, flattening them and adding decorative lines in the tops.

Bake 22 to 30 minutes or until golden brown. Transfer and let cool completely on a wire rack. Store the cookies in an airtight container in the refrigerator. For more options, read the "Storage Tips" section on page 19.

PEANUT BUTTER FRUIT SNACKS

{ COOL COOKIES FOR STRESSED-OUT DOGS }

1 c. rolled oats (the old-fashioned kind, not instant)

1 c. oat bran

$1/4$ c. dried cranberries

$1/4$ c. finely chopped peanuts

$1/4$ c. shredded coconut (unsweetened)

$1/4$ c. honey

$1/2$ c. peanut butter (unsalted)

CBD oil (see page 16 for dosage amounts)

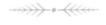

Mix all ingredients together. Drop the mixture by tablespoon into mini cupcake papers and place on a rimmed baking sheet or large plate. Put in the refrigerator for 15 minutes, or until set. Store the cookies in an airtight container in the refrigerator. For more options, read the "Storage Tips" section on page 19.

PUMPKIN SPICE COOKIES

{ A FUN FALL TREAT }

1 ½ c. oat flour
1 ½ c. brown rice flour
½ tsp. cinnamon
½ tsp. ground ginger
1 egg
3 tbsp. applesauce (unsweetened)
¾ c. canned pumpkin (or fresh, pureed pumpkin)
CBD oil (see page 16 for dosage amounts)
½ c. water (add slowly)

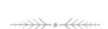

Preheat oven to 350°F. Combine all ingredients (except the water) together. Add water slowly and mix until a dough forms (if too dry, add more water; too wet, add a bit more flour). You may not need all the water if you reach a good consistency first. Line a cookie sheet with parchment paper (for easy cleanup). Spoon the mixture out with a tablespoon and place on the tray (they can be rather close together, as they don't grow much while cooking). These cookies will not rise or flatten, so if you want a flatter cookie, press each one down before baking.

Bake 18 to 25 minutes or until golden brown. Transfer and let cool completely on a wire rack. Store the cookies in an airtight container in the refrigerator. For more options, read the "Storage Tips" section on page 19.

OUT OF THE PATCH & INTO THE BOWL

Pumpkin is a nutritious and delicious food whose benefits can be reaped by including it in recipes that go well beyond the traditional holiday pie—and your dog shouldn't be getting any of that pie, anyway! Pumpkin is high in potassium and beta-carotene (a natural antioxidant) but low in calories, so when steamed and eaten in chunks or pureed, it's great for those watching their weight who want to enjoy a flavorful and filling veggie. A tablespoon or two of canned (or fresh) pumpkin added to their food will firm up your dog's stool if they have diarrhea or help loosen it if they're constipated (it's true, it works both ways). It's a miracle food!

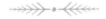

CHEWY GINGER MOLASSES COOKIES

{ GINGER SNAPS FOR YOUR PUP }

2 c. oat flour

2 c. brown rice flour

2 tsp. baking soda

2 tsp. ground ginger

1 tsp. cinnamon

1 tsp. ground cloves

1 egg

1/4 c. safflower oil

1/2 c. molasses (blackstrap or regular)

CBD oil (see page 16 for dosage amounts)

1/2 c. water (add slowly)

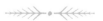

Preheat oven to 350°F. Combine all ingredients (except the water) together. Add water slowly and mix until a dough forms (if too dry, add more water; too wet, add a bit more flour). You may not need all the water if you reach a good consistency first. Spoon out the mixture and roll into balls (about 1" in diameter). Line a cookie sheet with parchment paper (for easy cleanup), and place the cookies on the sheet (they can be rather close together, as they don't grow much while cooking). These cookies will not rise or flatten, so if you want a flatter cookie, press each one down before baking.

Bake 22 to 30 minutes or until golden brown. Transfer and let cool completely on a wire rack. Store the cookies in an airtight container in the refrigerator. For more options, read the "Storage Tips" section on page 19.

GINGER

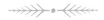

Besides having a smell that instantly transforms a house into a home (just as a dog does), ginger is a tasty and nutritious spice. It is especially beneficial for stomach upset.

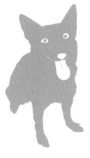

PUPPY PORRIDGE

{ OATMEAL COOKIES AS GOOD AS YOU REMEMBER }

1 1/2 c. oat flour
1 1/2 c. brown rice flour
1 tsp. baking powder
1/2 tsp. baking soda
1 c. rolled oats (the old-fashioned kind, not instant)
1/2 c. finely chopped peanuts (unsalted)
2 eggs
1/4 c. safflower oil
1/2 c. peanut butter (unsalted)
1/2 c. honey
1 tsp. vanilla
CBD oil (see page 16 for dosage amounts)
1/2 c. water (add slowly)

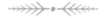

Preheat oven to 350°F. Combine all ingredients (except the water) together. Add water slowly and mix until a dough forms (if too dry, add more water; too wet, add a bit more flour). You may not need all the water if you reach a good consistency first. Line a cookie sheet with parchment paper (for easy cleanup), and spoon out the mixture and roll into balls (about 1" in diameter). Place on the sheet (they can be rather close together, as they don't grow much while cooking). Press each one down with your hand to flatten the cookies if you want; they don't flatten while cooking.

Bake 22 to 30 minutes or until golden brown. Transfer and let cool completely on a wire rack. Store the cookies in an airtight container in the refrigerator. For more options, read the "Storage Tips" section on page 19.

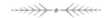

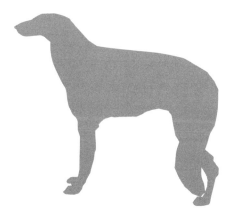

TROPICAL TREATS

{ THE FRUIT OF THE ISLANDS }

1 ½ c. oat flour
1 ½ c. brown rice flour
½ c. shredded coconut (unsweetened)
½ c. carob chips (do NOT substitute with chocolate)
1 egg
½ c. peanut butter (unsalted)
1 tsp. vanilla
CBD oil (see page 16 for dosage amounts)
½ c. water (add slowly)

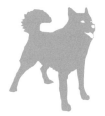

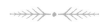

Preheat oven to 350°F. Combine all ingredients (except the water) together. Add water slowly and mix until a dough forms (if too dry, add more water; too wet, add a bit more flour). You may not need all the water if you reach a good consistency first. Line a cookie sheet with parchment paper (for easy cleanup), and spoon out the mixture and roll into balls (about 1" in diameter). Place on the sheet (they can be rather close together, as they don't grow much while cooking).

Bake 22 to 30 minutes or until golden brown. Transfer and let cool completely on a wire rack. Store the cookies in an airtight container in the refrigerator. For more options, read the "Storage Tips" section on page 19.

HONEY & OAT COOKIES

{ TASTY & TERRIFIC }

1 ½ c. brown rice flour

2 c. rolled oats (the old-fashioned kind, not instant)

1 egg

½ c. peanut butter (unsalted)

4 tbsp. applesauce (unsweetened)

¼ c. honey

CBD oil (see page 16 for dosage amounts)

¼ c. water (add slowly)

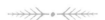

Preheat oven to 350°F. Combine all ingredients (except the water) together. Add water slowly and mix until a dough forms (if too dry, add more water; too wet, add a bit more flour). You may not need all the water if you reach a good consistency first. Line a cookie sheet with parchment paper (for easy cleanup), and spoon out the mixture and roll into balls (about 1" in diameter). Place on the sheet (they can be rather close together, as they don't grow much while cooking). Press each one down with your hand to flatten.

Bake 22 to 30 minutes or until golden brown. Transfer and let cool completely on a wire rack. Store the cookies in an airtight container in the refrigerator. For more options, read the "Storage Tips" section on page 19.

HIKER HELPER

{ TRAIL MIX FOR YOUR BEST PAL }

1 ¼ c. oat flour

1 ¼ c. brown rice flour

½ c. carob chips (do NOT substitute with chocolate)

½ c. granola (must NOT contain raisins)

½ c. shredded coconut (unsweetened)

½ c. dried cranberries

1 egg

¼ c. molasses (blackstrap or regular)

CBD oil (see page 16 for dosage amounts)

½ c. water (add slowly)

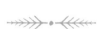

Preheat oven to 350°F. Combine all ingredients (except the water) together. Add water slowly and mix until a dough forms (if too dry, add more water; too wet, add a bit more flour). You may not need all the water if you reach a good consistency first. Line a cookie sheet with parchment paper (for easy cleanup), and spoon out the mixture and roll into balls (about 1" in diameter). Place on the sheet (they can be rather close together, as they don't grow much while cooking). Press each one down with your hand to flatten the cookies if you want; they don't flatten while cooking.

Bake 22 to 30 minutes or until golden brown. Transfer and let cool completely on a wire rack. Store the cookies in an airtight container in the refrigerator. For more options, read the "Storage Tips" section on page 19.

RID YOUR DOG'S PANTRY OF RAISINS

Though scientists haven't pinpointed what it is in raisins, exactly, that's toxic to dogs, they've seen enough cases of acute renal failure in dogs that have eaten various amounts of raisins (and grapes) to know that they contain something quite harmful. The veterinarian community is clear that raisins and grapes should not be fed to dogs.

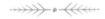

WHITE CHOCOLATE CHUNK COOKIES

{ DIDN'T YOU SAY CHOCOLATE WAS BAD?
NOT WHITE CHOCOLATE! }

1 ½ c. oat flour

1 ½ c. brown rice flour

½ c. dried cranberries

½ c. shredded coconut (unsweetened)

½ c. white chocolate chips or chunks

1 egg

CBD oil (see page 16 for dosage amounts)

½ c. water (add slowly)

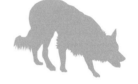

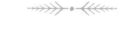

Preheat oven to 350°F. Combine all ingredients (except the water) together. Add water slowly and mix until a dough forms (if too dry, add more water; too wet, add a bit more flour). You may not need all the water if you reach a good consistency first. Line a cookie sheet with parchment paper (for easy cleanup), and spoon out the mixture and roll into balls (about 1" in diameter). Place on the sheet (they can be rather close together, as they don't grow much while cooking). Press each one down with your hand to flatten the cookies if you want; they don't flatten while cooking.

Bake 22 to 30 minutes or until golden brown. Transfer and let cool completely on a wire rack. Store the cookies in an airtight container in the refrigerator. For more options, read the "Storage Tips" section on page 19.

WHITE CHOCOLATE IN MODERATION

Why is white chocolate OK for dogs but milk or dark chocolate is an absolute no-no? Because white chocolate is really not chocolate at all. It is a mixture of cocoa butter, sugar, and milk. Originally made in Switzerland, it didn't become popular in the United States until the 1980s. Now it is marketed alongside regular chocolates as an equally creamy and sweet confection—and in limited quantities, it is a safe addition to canine cookies.

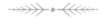

PIE IN THE SKY

{ APPLE PIE—A PERENNIAL HOLIDAY FAVORITE, NOW BITE-SIZE FOR YOUR PUP }

1 ½ c. oat flour
1 ½ c. brown rice flour
2 ½ tsp. cinnamon
½ c. oat bran
1 egg
½ c. applesauce (unsweetened)
2 tbsp. honey
CBD oil (see page 16 for dosage amounts)
¼ c. water (add slowly)

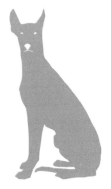

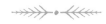

Preheat oven to 350°F. Combine all ingredients (except the water) together. Add water slowly and mix until a dough forms (if too dry, add more water; too wet, add a bit more flour). You may not need all the water if you reach a good consistency first. Line a cookie sheet with parchment paper (for easy cleanup), and spoon out the mixture and roll into balls (about 1" in diameter). Place on the sheet (they can be rather close together, as they don't grow much while cooking). Press each one down with your hand to flatten the cookies if you want; they don't flatten while cooking.

Bake 22 to 30 minutes or until golden brown. Transfer and let cool completely on a wire rack. Store the cookies in an airtight container in the refrigerator. For more options, read the "Storage Tips" section on page 19.

AN APPLE A DAY

You know the old saying "An apple a day keeps the doctor away"? The same, thankfully, can be said for dogs. Apples that have been thoroughly washed, have had the stems and seeds removed, and have been cut up into slices or chunks make great healthy snacks for dogs. Apples have numerous health benefits.

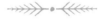

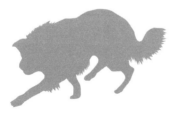

BERRY TASTY TREATS
{ LITTLE BITES OF BLUEBERRY GOODNESS }

1 ½ c. oat flour
1 ½ c. brown rice flour
½ c. frozen blueberries (or fresh)
1 egg
½ c. peanut butter (unsalted)
CBD oil (see page 16 for dosage amounts)
½ c. water (add slowly)

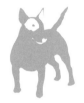

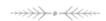

Preheat oven to 350°F. Combine all ingredients (except the water) together. Add water slowly and mix until a dough forms (if too dry, add more water; too wet, add a bit more flour). You may not need all the water if you reach a good consistency first. Line a cookie sheet with parchment paper (for easy cleanup), and spoon out the mixture and roll into balls (about 1" in diameter). Place on the sheet (they can be rather close together, as they don't grow much while cooking). Press each one down with your hand to flatten the cookies if you want; they don't flatten while cooking.

Bake 22 to 30 minutes or until golden brown. Transfer and let cool completely on a wire rack. Store the cookies in an airtight container in the refrigerator. For more options, read the "Storage Tips" section on page 19.

B-OAT-LOADS OF BANANAS

{ PEANUT BUTTER BANANA DROPS }

1 ½ c. oat flour

1 ½ c. brown rice flour

½ c. peanut butter (unsalted)

½ c. rolled oats (the old-fashioned kind, not instant)

1 egg

½ c. bananas (mashed and pureed)

CBD oil (see page 16 for dosage amounts)

½ c. water (add slowly)

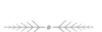

Preheat oven to 350°F. Combine all ingredients (except the water) together. Add water slowly and mix until a dough forms (if too dry, add more water; too wet, add a bit more flour). You may not need all the water if you reach a good consistency first. Line a cookie sheet with parchment paper (for easy cleanup), and spoon out the mixture and roll into balls (about 1" in diameter). Place on the sheet (they can be rather close together, as they don't grow much while cooking). Press each one down with your hand to flatten the cookies if you want; they don't flatten while cooking.

Bake 22 to 30 minutes or until golden brown. Transfer and let cool completely on a wire rack. Store the cookies in an airtight container in the refrigerator. For more options, read the "Storage Tips" section on page 19.

PEANUT BUTTER CRUNCH COOKIES

{ CLUSTERS OF PEANUT BUTTER GOODNESS }

1 ½ c. oat flour

1 ½ c. brown rice flour

½ c. finely chopped peanuts (unsalted)

½ c. shredded coconut (unsweetened)

½ c. rolled oats (the old-fashioned kind, not instant)

2 eggs

¼ c. molasses (blackstrap or regular)

½ c. peanut butter

CBD oil (see page 16 for dosage amounts)

½ c. water (add slowly)

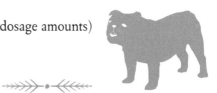

Preheat oven to 350°F. Combine all ingredients (except the water) together. Add water slowly and mix until a dough forms (if too dry, add more water; too wet, add a bit more flour). You may not need all the water if you reach a good consistency first. Line a cookie sheet with parchment paper (for easy cleanup), and spoon out the mixture and roll into balls (about 1" in diameter). Place on the sheet (they can be rather close together, as they don't grow much while cooking).

These cookies will not rise or flatten, so if you want a flatter cookie, press each one down before baking.

Bake 22 to 30 minutes or until golden brown. Transfer and let cool completely on a wire rack. Store the cookies in an airtight container in the refrigerator. For more options, read the "Storage Tips" section on page 19.

COCONUT

Coconut is an excellent source of lauric acid, manganese, iron, phosphorus, and potassium. It is a rich protein source that supports skin and coat health. It also supports the healthy function of the thyroid and the immune system, as well as gastrointestinal, digestive, cell, and bone function.

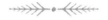

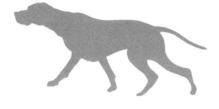

MUD TRACKS

{ THE ONLY ACCEPTABLE KIND IN THE HOUSE }

1 ½ c. oat flour
1 ½ c. brown rice flour
¼ c. carob powder (do NOT substitute with chocolate)
½ c. carob chips (do NOT substitute with chocolate)
1 egg
½ c. peanut butter (unsalted)
1 tbsp. honey
CBD oil (see page 16 for dosage amounts)
⅔ c. water (add slowly)

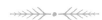

Preheat oven to 350°F. Combine all ingredients (except the water) together. Add water slowly and mix until a dough forms (if too dry, add more water; too wet, add a bit more flour). You may not need all the water if you reach a good consistency first. Line a cookie sheet with parchment paper (for easy cleanup), and spoon out the mixture and roll into balls (about 1" in diameter). Place on the sheet (they can be rather close together, as they don't grow much while cooking). These cookies will not rise or flatten, so if you want a flatter cookie, press each one down before baking.

Bake 22 to 30 minutes or until golden brown. Transfer and let cool completely on a wire rack. Store the cookies in an airtight container in the refrigerator. For more options, read the "Storage Tips" section on page 19.

Note: Carob powder and carob chips are generally carried in all health food stores or are available online.

PEANUT BUTTER

As oily as it looks, peanut butter is high in monounsaturated fats—the kind that protect against heart disease. Grinding your own (organic) nuts yields a butter of exceptional flavor and avoids the sugars and salts that are often added to commercial varieties. Peanuts are an excellent source of protein as well.

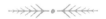

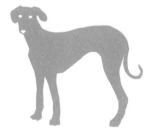

COCO LOCO

{ COCONUT-COVERED BALLS OF GOODNESS }

1 ½ c. oat flour
1 ½ c. brown rice flour
1 c. shredded coconut (unsweetened)
1 tsp. cinnamon
1 egg
1 tsp. vanilla
CBD oil (see page 16 for dosage amounts)
½ c. coconut milk (add slowly)

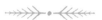

Preheat oven to 350°F. Combine all ingredients (except the coconut milk) together. Add coconut milk slowly and mix until a dough forms (if too dry, add more coconut milk; too wet, add a bit more flour). You may not need all the coconut milk if you reach a good consistency first. Line a cookie sheet with parchment paper (for easy cleanup). Spoon out the mixture and roll into balls (about 1" in diameter) in the coconut. Place the cookies on the sheet (they can be rather close together, as they don't grow much while cooking).

Bake 22 to 30 minutes or until golden brown. Transfer and let cool completely on a wire rack. Store the cookies in an airtight container in the refrigerator. For more options, read the "Storage Tips" section on page 19.

BUDDY'S NUTTY NOMS

{ YOUR DOG WILL GO NUTS FOR THIS ONE }

1 ½ c. oat flour
1 ½ c. brown rice flour
½ c. finely ground peanuts
1 egg
½ c. molasses (blackstap or regular)
1 tsp. vanilla
CBD oil (see page 16 for dosage amounts)
½ c. water (add slowly)

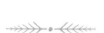

Preheat oven to 350°F. Combine all ingredients (except the water) together. Add water slowly and mix until a dough forms (if too dry, add more water; too wet, add a bit more flour). You may not need all the water if you reach a good consistency first. Line a cookie sheet with parchment paper (for easy cleanup), and spoon out the mixture and roll into balls (about 1" in diameter). Place on the sheet (they can be rather close together, as they don't grow much while cooking). These cookies will not rise or flatten, so if you want a flatter cookie, press each one down before baking.

Bake 22 to 30 minutes or until golden brown. Transfer and let cool completely on a wire rack. Store the cookies in an airtight container in the refrigerator. For more options, read the "Storage Tips" section on page 19.

PEPPER-PRINTS

{ THESE ARE SURE TO STRAIGHTEN THEIR TAIL- & FRESHEN THEIR BREATH }

1 ½ c. oat flour
1 ½ c. brown rice flour
½ c. dried mint
¼ tsp. peppermint oil
1 egg
CBD oil (see page 16 for dosage amounts)
½ c. water (add slowly)

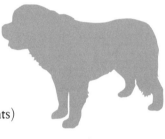

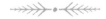

Preheat oven to 350°F. Combine all ingredients (except the water) together. Add water slowly and mix until a dough forms (if too dry, add more water; too wet, add a bit more flour). You may not need all the water if you reach a good consistency first. Line a cookie sheet with parchment paper (for easy cleanup), and spoon out the mixture and roll into balls (about 1" in diameter). Place on the sheet (they can be rather close together, as they don't grow much while cooking). These cookies will not rise or flatten, so if you want a flatter cookie, press each one down before baking.

Bake 22 to 30 minutes or until golden brown. Transfer and let cool completely on a wire rack. Store the cookies in an airtight container in the refrigerator. For more options, read the "Storage Tips" section on page 19.

PEPPERMINT

Mints have long been associated with aiding in digestive upset, and this is true for dogs as well as people. They have the added benefit of being able to freshen breath. A double whammy for dogs!

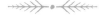

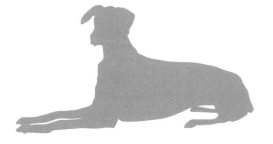

CAN'T CATCH ME

{ I'M THE GINGERBREAD MAN }

1 ½ c. oat flour
1 ½ c. brown rice flour
1 tsp. baking powder
1 tsp. ground ginger
1 tsp. cinnamon
½ tsp. baking soda
1 egg
¼ c. safflower oil
½ c. molasses (blackstrap or regular)
¼ c. peanut butter (unsalted)
1 tbsp. apple cider vinegar
CBD oil (see page 16 for dosage amounts)
½ c. water (add slowly)

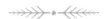

Preheat oven to 350°F. Combine all ingredients (except the water) together. Add water slowly and mix until a dough forms (if too dry, add more water; too wet, add a bit more flour). You may not need all the water if you reach a good consistency first. Line a cookie sheet with parchment paper (for easy cleanup), and spoon out the mixture and roll into balls (about 1" in diameter). Place on the sheet (they can be rather close together, as they don't grow much while cooking). These cookies will not rise or flatten, so if you want a flatter cookie, press each one down before baking.

Bake 22 to 30 minutes or until golden brown. Transfer and let cool completely on a wire rack. Store the cookies in an airtight container in the refrigerator. For more options, read the "Storage Tips" section on page 19.

APPLE CIDER VINEGAR

It seems you can't go wrong giving your dog apple cider vinegar — inside and out! The easiest way to introduce it to your dog's regular diet is to put a tiny amount in the water bowl. As they become used to the taste, increase the amount ever so gradually until you are adding about a teaspoon a day in the water. ACV is good for arthritis, allergies, itchy skin, correcting pH levels, eliminating tear stains around the eyes, fighting fleas and other pests, and so much more!

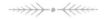

THESE BERRIES ARE BANANAS

{ B-A-N-A-N-A-S, WITH STRAWBERRIES }

1 ½ c. oat flour
1 ½ c. brown rice flour
1 tsp. cinnamon
1 tsp. honey
1 egg
½ c. strawberries (fresh or frozen, mashed and pureed)
½ c. bananas (mashed and pureed)
CBD oil (see page 16 for dosage amounts)
½ c. water (add slowly)

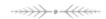

Preheat oven to 350°F. Combine all ingredients (except the water) together. Add water slowly and mix until a dough forms (if too dry, add more water; too wet, add a bit more flour). You may not need all the water if you reach a good consistency first.

Line a cookie sheet with parchment paper (for easy cleanup), and spoon out the mixture and roll into balls (about 1" in diameter). Place on the sheet (they can be rather close together, as they don't grow much while cooking). These cookies will not rise or flatten, so if you want a flatter cookie, press each one down before baking.

Bake 22 to 30 minutes or until golden brown. Transfer and let cool completely on a wire rack. Store the cookies in an airtight container in the refrigerator. For more options, read the "Storage Tips" section on page 19.

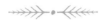

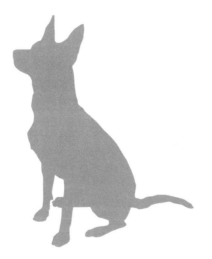

CHAPTER 5

EASYGOING EXTRAVAGANCE

For those with richer tastes

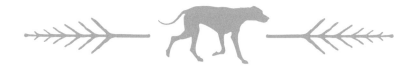

This collection of sweets strays from the path of the others by exploring combinations that are both indulgent and delightful. Some are simple, some are sinful. Like a stroll down easy street, where the riches of the world entice you, these goodies will have your dog pining by the cookie jar. This is also where you'll find recipes for cakes, cupcakes, and muffins, as well as icing options. Let your dog experience the ease and comfort that these decadent treats will offer.

CRUNCHY CANTUCCI

{ STRAIGHT FROM THE MOST UPSCALE CAFE }

$1/2$ c. bananas

2 $1/2$ c. oat flour

2 $1/2$ c. brown rice flour

2 tsp. baking powder

$1/2$ tsp baking soda

2 eggs

1 tsp. vanilla

1 tbsp. honey

$1/4$ c. finely chopped peanuts

CBD oil (see page 16 for dosage amounts)

A small container of water

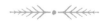

Preheat oven to 325°F. Mash bananas and puree in a food processor.

Combine all ingredients together in a food processor (or by hand in a bowl). Add 1 tbsp. of water at a time until the dough reaches a workable consistency. Once the dough is formed, knead together by hand for several minutes on a lightly floured surface. Separate into two logs about 12" long by 4" wide and 1" high. Line a cookie sheet with parchment paper (for easy cleanup), and place the cantucci on the sheet (they can be rather close together, as they don't grow much while cooking).

Bake for 30 minutes. Remove and let cool on the baking sheet for 10 minutes. Slice pieces $\frac{1}{2}$" thick. Bake an additional 20 minutes. Remove and place on a wire rack to cool completely. Store the cookies in an airtight container in the refrigerator. For more options, read the "Storage Tips" section on page 19.

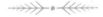

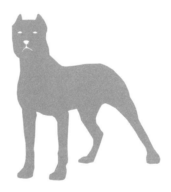

CRANBERRY DELICIOUS

{ A PERFECT TEA-TIME TREAT }

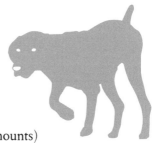

$^1/_2$ c. dried cranberries

1 $^1/_2$ c. oat flour

1 $^1/_2$ c. brown rice flour

2 tsp. baking powder

$^1/_2$ c. peanut butter (unsalted)

$^1/_4$ c. safflower oil

1 egg

CBD oil (see page 16 for dosage amounts)

$^1/_2$ c. water (add slowly)

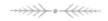

Preheat oven to 350°F. Set cranberries aside for later. Combine all ingredients (except the water) together. Add water slowly and mix until a dough forms (if too dry, add more water; too wet, add a bit more flour). You may not need all the water if you reach a good consistency first. Once combined, gently stir in cranberries by hand. Line a cookie sheet with parchment paper (for easy cleanup), and scoop out heaping spoonfuls (they can be rather close together, as they don't grow much while cooking).

Bake 25 to 30 minutes or until a toothpick inserted into the center of the cookie comes out cleanly. Remove from the oven and let cool completely. Store the cookies in an airtight container in the refrigerator. For more options, read the "Storage Tips" section on page 19.

BERRY, BERRY YUMMY

Several of the recipes in this chapter call for various berries, including cranberries, blueberries, and strawberries. Wonder no longer: all are safe for dogs. Berries are natural antioxidants; in fact, recent studies have shown that blueberries are especially rich in them. Cranberries are known for relieving urinary tract infections and promoting uterine health. Berries also contain lots of vitamin C. They are naturally sweet and tasty, and dogs really enjoy them. They can be served fresh, frozen, or dried.

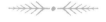

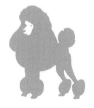

SWEETIE PIE

{ SWEET POTATO PASTRIES }

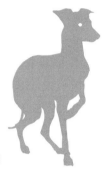

FOR THE DOUGH:

1 c. oat flour

1/2 c. brown rice flour

1/4 c. safflower oil

1/4 c. water

1 egg

CBD oil (see page 16 for dosage amounts)

1/2 c. water (add slowly)

FOR THE FILLING:

1 c. cooked, mashed sweet potato (or pumpkin)

1 tsp. cinnamon

1 tbsp. honey

1 tsp. ground cloves

1 egg

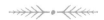

Preheat oven to 350°F. Combine all dough ingredients (except the water) together. Add water slowly and mix until a dough forms (if too dry, add more water; too wet, add a bit more flour). You may not need all the water if you reach a good consistency first. Roll out on a lightly floured surface to $\frac{1}{4}$" thickness. Use a 2" circle cookie cutter (or top of a glass, if you don't have a circle cookie cutter) to cut into shapes. Thoroughly spray cooking spray into the cups of a mini muffin pan and press each circle down into the cups.

Combine all the filling ingredients together and mix thoroughly. Scoop even amounts into each of the crusts in the muffin pan.

Bake for 25 to 30 minutes or until the edges of the crust are golden brown. Transfer and let cool completely on a wire rack. Store the treats in an airtight container in the refrigerator. For more options, read the "Storage Tips" section on page 19.

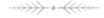

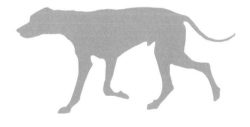

APPLE-Y EVER AFTER

{ APPLE SPICE MUFFINS }

1 ½ c. oat flour
1 ½ c. brown rice flour
1 tbsp. baking powder
1 tsp. cinnamon
2 eggs
¾ c. honey
1 c. applesauce (unsweetened)
¼ c. safflower oil
CBD oil (see page 16 for dosage amounts)

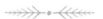

Preheat oven to 350°F. Combine all ingredients together and mix thoroughly. Place cupcake papers into a muffin pan. Spoon the mixture evenly into the papers, coming close to the top.

Bake 18 to 22 minutes or until a toothpick inserted into the center comes out clean. Transfer and let cool completely on a wire rack. Store in an airtight container in the refrigerator. For more options, read the "Storage Tips" section on page 19.

ROCKIN' THE OAT

{ SEAWORTHY BERRY OAT BITES }

1 ½ c. oat flour

1 c. rolled oats (the old-fashioned kind, not instant)

¼ tsp. baking soda

⅔ c. honey

¼ c. safflower oil

2 ½ c. blueberries (fresh or frozen)

CBD oil (see page 16 for dosage amounts)

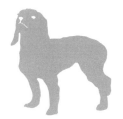

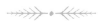

Preheat oven to 350°F. Combine all ingredients (except the blueberries) together and mix thoroughly. Separate the mixture in half. Lightly grease a muffin pan with cooking spray and press half of the mixture into the bottom of the muffin cups. Evenly spread the berries on top. Then sprinkle the remaining crumb mixture on top of the berries.

Bake for 30 to 35 minutes or until top is golden brown. Transfer and let cool completely on a wire rack. Store in an airtight container in the refrigerator. For more options, read the "Storage Tips" section on page 19.

BARKING BROWNIES

{ WITH CAROB—THE PERFECT BROWNIE }

FOR THE BROWNIES:

2 c. oat flour

1 tsp. baking powder

5 tbsp. carob powder (do NOT substitute with chocolate)

2 eggs

3/4 c. honey

1/4 c. safflower oil

1/2 c. nonfat vanilla yogurt (or use nonfat plain yogurt
   and add 1 tsp. vanilla)

CBD oil (see page 16 for dosage amounts)

FOR THE FROSTING:

8-oz. package low-fat cream cheese (at room temperature)

1/4 c. carob powder (do NOT substitute with chocolate)

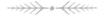

Preheat oven to 350°F. Combine all brownie ingredients together. Lightly grease a 9" square pan and pour the mixture in.

Bake 30 to 35 minutes or until sides of brownies seem to be loosening from the pan. Cool completely in the pan.

In a separate bowl, mix together frosting ingredients. Spread frosting on top of cooled brownies. Slice into individual-sized portions. Store in an airtight container in the refrigerator. For more options, read the "Storage Tips" section on page 19.

YOGURT? YOU BET!

Yogurt is another beneficial food that has been around forever. It is an excellent source of protein, and because it has less milk sugar, it is easily digested, even by lactose-intolerant animals. It also contains beneficial bacteria that support the digestive and immune systems, and it is a great source of calcium. A tablespoon or so of organic, plain, low-fat yogurt can benefit your dog in many ways. It is especially helpful when your dog is on antibiotics, as it restores some of the beneficial bacteria that the antibiotics randomly strip away or break down.

BOUNTIFUL BANANA BARS

{ BANANA PUMPKIN GOODNESS }

2 c. bananas
2 c. pumpkin (canned or fresh)
1 ½ c. oat flour
1 ½ c. brown rice flour
1 c. rolled oats (the old-fashioned kind, not instant)
1 tsp. cinnamon
2 eggs
¼ c. safflower oil
½ c. molasses (blackstrap or regular)
CBD oil (see page 16 for dosage amounts)

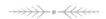

Preheat oven to 350°F. Mash and puree the bananas and pumpkin, if necessary.

Combine all ingredients together until thoroughly mixed. Lightly grease a 9" square pan and pour the mixture in.

Bake 30 to 35 minutes or until top appears golden brown and sides begin to slightly loosen from the pan. Transfer and let cool completely on a wire rack. Once cool, slice into individual-sized squares. Store in an airtight container in the refrigerator. For more options, read the "Storage Tips" section on page 19.

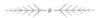

BIRTHDAY PARTY

{ CELEBRATE THAT SPECIAL DAY WITH CAKE }

FOR THE CAKE:

2 c. oat flour

$^{1}/_{2}$ c. carob powder (do NOT substitute with chocolate)

1 tsp. baking powder

2 eggs

$^{1}/_{4}$ c. safflower oil

$^{1}/_{2}$ c. honey

1 c. nonfat vanilla yogurt (or use nonfat plain yogurt
    and add 1 tsp. vanilla)

CBD oil (see page 16 for dosage amounts)

FOR THE ICING:

8-oz. package nonfat cream cheese (at room temperature)

1 tbsp. honey

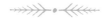

Preheat oven to 350°F. Combine all cake ingredients together and mix thoroughly. Lightly grease a 6" round cake pan (preferably a 3" tall pan, but 2" is fine too) and pour the mixture in.

Bake 30 to 35 minutes or until a toothpick inserted in the center of the cake comes out clean. Transfer and let cool completely on a wire rack.

In a separate bowl, combine icing ingredients. Once the cake is completely cooled, decorate with the icing. Store in an airtight container in the refrigerator. For more options, read the "Storage Tips" section on page 19.

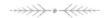

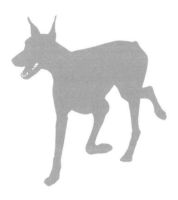

BLONDIE BARS

{ ...THEN IT'S GOT TO BE A BLONDIE! }

2 c. oat flour

1 tsp. baking powder

2 eggs

$\frac{1}{2}$ c. honey

$\frac{1}{4}$ c. peanut butter (unsalted)

$\frac{1}{4}$ c. safflower oil

$\frac{1}{2}$ c. plain or vanilla nonfat yogurt

CBD oil (see page 16 for dosage amounts)

1 c. carob chips (do NOT substitute with chocolate)

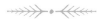

Preheat oven to 350°F. Combine all ingredients (except the carob chips) together in a large bowl. Stir in carob chips by hand until evenly mixed. Lightly grease a square 9" pan and pour the mixture in.

Bake 30 to 35 minutes or until the sides loosen from the pan and the top appears golden brown. Transfer and let cool completely on a wire rack. Once cool, slice into individual-sized portions. Store in an airtight container in the refrigerator. For more options, read the "Storage Tips" section on page 19.

ICING, ICING BABY
{ GREAT FOR COOKIES & GIFT GIVING }

....

This will set and be a hard icing, so you can box up the treats if desired. You can use this on top of any of the treats in this book.

FOR CAROB ICING (DARK BROWN):
1 c. unsweetened carob chips (do NOT substitute with chocolate)

FOR WHITE OR COLORED ICING:
2 c. yogurt coating chips
Natural liquid food colorings

You can add CBD oil to this recipe if desired (see page 16 for dosage amounts), but be careful to consider how much CBD is already in any treat you may be topping with this icing. These chips need to be heated in a double boiler (over low heat) on the oven or in the microwave. Once soft, you can either dip your treats into them, or if you're feeling ambitious, use a pastry bag with a decorating tip to ice the tops of the cookies. If the carob or yogurt chips are too thick to work with when melted, you can add a splash of safflower oil to help thin it out, but be careful, because if you add too much it won't harden again when it cools.

Carob chips, natural food colorings, and yogurt chips should be available in any health food store or the natural aisle in your local supermarket. If you are having trouble finding them, there are some great places to order them online; one site is www.barryfarm.com

BAKING CARE OF BUSINESS

{ BLUEBERRY MUFFINS—A FAVORITE TREAT FOR ALL }

2 c. oat flour

2 tsp. baking powder

1 tsp. cinnamon

1 tsp. baking soda

2 c. blueberries (fresh or frozen)

3 eggs

$\frac{1}{4}$ c. honey

$\frac{1}{4}$ c. safflower oil

CBD oil (see page 16 for dosage amounts)

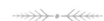

Preheat oven to 350°F. Combine all ingredients together and mix thoroughly. Place cupcake papers into a mini muffin pan (or a regular muffin pan). Spoon the mixture evenly into the papers, coming almost to the top (the mix will not rise very much).

Bake 10 to 15 minutes if using the mini muffin pan, or 22 to 27 minutes if using a regular-sized muffin pan. Muffins are done when a toothpick inserted into the center comes out clean. Transfer and let cool completely on a wire rack. Store in an airtight container in the refrigerator. For more options, read the "Storage Tips" section on page 19.

ICING THIS ICING'S PRAISES

{ CAN BE USED ON ANY TREAT }

This will be soft and require refrigeration, but it is a more natural "icing" if you do not want to use the carob or yogurt chips. You can use this on top of any of the treats in this book.

8-oz. package of nonfat cream cheese
2 tbsp. honey
Natural liquid food colorings

You can add CBD oil to this recipe if desired (see page 16 for dosage amounts), but be careful to consider how much CBD is already in any treat you may be topping with this icing. Let the cream cheese warm to room temperature, and then mix the cream cheese and honey in a bowl. If you want to add color, put in a few drops of a natural food coloring at this time. You can find natural liquid food coloring in most health food stores. Spread the icing over your cookies and store in a covered container in the refrigerator. For more options, read the "Storage Tips" section on page 19.

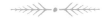

FRO-YO

....

BANANA, STRAWBERRY, APPLE:
1 mashed and pureed banana
1 c. plain nonfat yogurt
1 c. pureed strawberries
2 c. apple juice

BLUEBERRY HONEY:
2 c. nonfat plain yogurt
1 c. pureed blueberries (fresh or frozen)
2 tbsp. honey

SAVORY CHICKEN CRANBERRY:
2 c. nonfat plain yogurt
2 c. chicken broth
1 c. pureed cranberries (fresh or dried)
1 tsp. rosemary

PEANUT BUTTER BACON:
2 c. plain nonfat yogurt
1 c. peanut butter (unsalted)
2 slices bacon (precooked, drained, and finely ground)

PUMPKIN PIE:

2 c. nonfat plain yogurt

1 c. canned pumpkin (fresh is always fine too)

1 tsp. cinnamon

2 tbsp. honey

CAROB CHIP CRUNCH:

2 c. nonfat plain yogurt

1 c. carob chips (do NOT substitute with chocolate)

2 tbsp. peanut butter (unsalted)

2 tbsp. honey

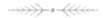

Combine all ingredients (from respective recipe) together with CBD oil (see page 16 for dosage amounts) and whisk thoroughly. Pour the mixture into an ice cube tray. Freeze until solid (at least 4 hours).

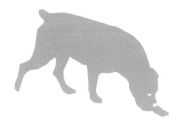

A-PEELING
PEANUT CUPCAKES
{ KEEP THAT FIGURE LEAN & MEAN! }

FOR THE CUPCAKES:

3 bananas

2 c. oat flour

2 tsp. baking powder

$^1\!/_2$ tsp. baking soda

1 tsp. cinnamon

$^1\!/_2$ c. finely chopped peanuts

3 eggs

$^1\!/_4$ c. honey

$^1\!/_4$ c. safflower oil

CBD oil (see page 16 for dosage amounts)

FOR THE ICING (OPTIONAL):

1 c. banana, mashed and pureed

8-oz. package nonfat cream cheese (at room temperature)

1 tsp. vanilla

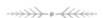

Preheat oven to 350°F. Peel, mash, and puree the bananas (for the cupcakes).

Combine all cupcake ingredients together in a large bowl. Place cupcake papers in a mini muffin pan and spoon the mixture into the cups evenly. Fill almost to the top of the papers as the cupcakes don't rise very much.

Bake 12 to 15 minutes or until a toothpick inserted in the center of a cupcake comes out clean. Transfer and let cool completely on a wire rack.

In a separate bowl, combine icing ingredients together and mix thoroughly. Decorate the mini cupcakes. Store in an airtight container in the refrigerator. For more options, read the "Storage Tips" section on page 19.

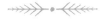

SUMMER SQUASH BISCUITS

{ DOGS ENJOY THEIR VERSION OF ZUCCHINI BREAD AS MUCH AS PEOPLE DO }

2 c. zucchini

2 c. oat flour

2 tsp. baking powder

$^{1}/_{2}$ tsp. baking soda

1 tsp. cinnamon

3 eggs

1 tsp. vanilla

$^{3}/_{4}$ c. honey

$^{1}/_{4}$ c. safflower oil

CBD oil (see page 16 for dosage amounts)

$^{1}/_{2}$ c. finely chopped peanuts (optional)

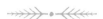

Preheat oven to 325°F. Cook and slice zucchini, and then puree in a food processor.

Combine all ingredients together and mix thoroughly. Lightly grease a mini loaf pan (or use a regular muffin pan with cupcake papers placed in it). Spoon the mixture evenly into the pan, coming close to the top (the mix will not rise very much).

Bake 20 to 25 minutes (with either pan). Bread is done when a toothpick inserted into the center comes out clean. Transfer and let cool completely on a wire rack. Store in an airtight container in the refrigerator. For more options, read the "Storage Tips" section on page 19.

ZUCCHINI'S SO GOOD

Zucchini is one of several squashes that were a mainstay of Native American diets for centuries. These large, green vegetables are loaded with folate and potassium. Their peels are rich in beta-carotene and should always be included in any recipe featuring this versatile squash.

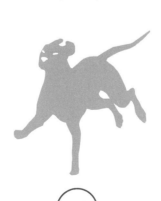

179

PUPNUT BRITTLE

{ DOGS WILL BE BEGGING FOR MORE! }

3 c. brown rice flour

1 tsp. cinnamon

1 egg

½ c. honey

¼ c. molasses (blackstrap or regular)

½ c. peanut butter (unsalted)

¼ c. safflower oil

CBD oil (see page 16 for dosage amounts)

1 c. finely chopped peanuts (unsalted)

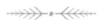

Preheat oven to 325°F. Combine all ingredients (except the chopped peanuts) in a food processor until completely mixed. It should form a stiff dough. Lightly grease a jelly roll pan and press the dough into the pan. Place plastic wrap or parchment paper over the pan and smooth down the mixture to ¼" thick. Remove and discard wrap or paper.

Press the chopped peanuts into the mixture. Use a knife to score the dough into individual-sized portions.

Bake 30 to 40 minutes or until the edges are golden brown. Cool completely in the pan on a wire rack. Once cool, break apart using the scored lines. Store in a loosely covered container at room temperature. For more options, read the "Storage Tips" section on page 19.

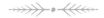

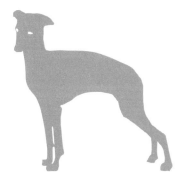

POP-UP PASTRIES

{ NO TOASTER NEEDED FOR THESE SNACKS! }

FOR THE DOUGH:

1 c. oat flour

½ c. brown rice flour

1 egg

¼ c. safflower oil

CBD oil (see page 16 for dosage amounts)

¼ c. water (add slowly)

FOR THE FILLING:

½ c. blueberries (fresh or frozen)

½ c. diced strawberries (fresh or frozen)

1 tsp. vanilla

½ c. peanut butter (unsalted)

1 egg

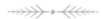

Preheat oven to 350°F. Combine all dough ingredients (except the water) together. Add water slowly and mix until a dough forms (if too dry, add more water; too wet, add a bit more flour). You may not need all the water if you reach a good consistency first. Roll out on a lightly floured surface to ¼" thickness. Use a 2" circle cookie cutter (or top of a glass, if you don't have a circle cookie cutter) to cut into shapes. Thoroughly spray cooking spray into the cups of a mini muffin pan and press each circle down into the cups. Combine all the filling ingredients together and mix thoroughly. Scoop even amounts into each of the crusts in the muffin pan.

Bake for 25 to 30 minutes or until the edges of the crust are golden brown. Transfer and let cool completely on a wire rack. Store the treats in an airtight container in the refrigerator. For more options, read the "Storage Tips" section on page 19.

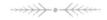

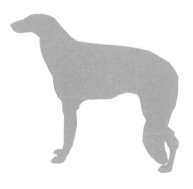

ALMOST-CHOCOLATE CUPCAKES

{ THE DOG-SAFE VERSION OF A CHOCOLATE CUPCAKE }

1 c. oat flour

1 c. brown rice flour

2 tsp. baking soda

$^{1}/_{2}$ tsp. baking powder

$^{1}/_{4}$ c. carob powder (do NOT substitute with chocolate)

1 egg

2 tbsp. honey

$^{1}/_{4}$ c. safflower oil

$^{1}/_{2}$ c. plain nonfat yogurt

CBD oil (see page 16 for dosage amounts)

$^{1}/_{4}$ c. water

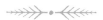

Preheat oven to 350°F. Combine all ingredients together and mix thoroughly. Place cupcake papers into a mini muffin pan (or a regular muffin pan). Spoon the mixture evenly into the papers, coming close to the top of the papers (the mix will not rise very much).

Bake 10 to 15 minutes if using the mini muffin pan, or 20 to 25 minutes if using a regular-sized muffin pan. Cupcakes are done when a toothpick inserted into the center comes out clean. Transfer and let cool completely on a wire rack. Store in an airtight container in the refrigerator. For more options, read the "Storage Tips" section on page 19.

Note: These can be iced with one of the icing recipes described in earlier recipes. We recommend the soft icing recipe on page 173, and if you're feeling extra adventurous, you can add toppings to the top of the icing. Some good ideas would be ground peanuts, carob chips, granola (make sure it is raisin free), sliced bananas, etc. The possibilities are endless.

TRAIL BLAZER

{ TRAIL MIX WITHOUT THE BAG }

....

2 c. oat flour

1 tsp. baking powder

$\frac{1}{2}$ c. peanut butter (unsalted)

$\frac{1}{2}$ c. rolled oats (the old-fashioned kind, not instant)

$\frac{1}{2}$ c. finely chopped peanuts (unsalted)

$\frac{1}{2}$ c. shredded coconut (unsweetened)

$\frac{1}{2}$ c. dried cranberries

$\frac{1}{2}$ c. carob chips (do NOT substitute with chocolate)

2 eggs

$\frac{1}{2}$ c. honey

1 tsp. vanilla

$\frac{1}{4}$ c. safflower oil

CBD oil (see page 16 for dosage amounts)

1 c. water

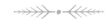

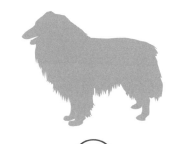

Preheat oven to 350°F. Combine all ingredients together and mix thoroughly. Lightly grease a 9" square baking pan and pour the mixture into it.

Bake for 30 to 35 minutes or until top is golden brown. Transfer and let cool completely on a wire rack. Once cool, slice into individual-sized portions. Store in an airtight container in the refrigerator. For more options, read the "Storage Tips" section on page 19.

A TASTE OF THE TROPICS

The Coconut Research Center in Colorado has this to say about the benefits of coconut: "Coconut is highly nutritious and rich in fiber, vitamins, and minerals. It is classified as a 'functional food' because it provides many health benefits beyond its nutritional content. Coconut oil is of special interest because it possesses healing properties far beyond that of any other dietary oil and is extensively used in traditional medicine among Asian and Pacific populations. Pacific Islanders consider coconut oil to be the cure for all illness. The coconut palm is so highly valued by them as both a source of food and medicine that it is called 'The Tree of Life.' Only recently has modern medical science unlocked the secrets to coconut's amazing healing powers." Use unsweetened coconut for dogs, and consider serving it to them more often!

PUP-KIN MUFFINS

{ DOGS LOVE THE TASTE OF PUMPKIN,
& IT HELPS THEIR DIGESTIVE SYSTEM TOO }

2 c. oat flour
2 tsp. baking powder
2 tsp. cinnamon
$\frac{1}{2}$ tsp. baking soda
$\frac{1}{2}$ tsp. ground cloves
3 eggs
$\frac{3}{4}$ c. honey
$\frac{1}{4}$ c. safflower oil
15-oz. can pumpkin (or fresh pureed pumpkin)
CBD oil (see page 16 for dosage amounts)

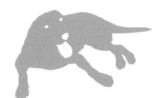

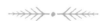

Preheat oven to 350°F. Combine all ingredients together and mix thoroughly. Place cupcake papers into a mini muffin pan (or a regular muffin pan). Spoon the mixture evenly into the papers, coming close to the top of the papers (the mix will not rise very much).

Bake 10 to 15 minutes if using the mini muffin pan, or 22 to 27 minutes if using a regular-sized muffin pan. Muffins are done when a toothpick inserted into the center comes out clean. Transfer and let cool completely on a wire rack. Store in an airtight container in the refrigerator. For more options, read the "Storage Tips" section on page 19.

Note: Throwing a party for your dog with all their friends in attendance and want to make a larger cake? This is a great recipe for that, along with our other soft muffin recipes. Instead of using a cupcake pan, just pour the batter into a 6" cake pan (if you have any left over, you can even make a few muffins out of it). Keep in mind that the cake will take a lot longer to cook, so you can anticipate more like 35 to 40 minutes for it to finish cooking. The cake will be done when a toothpick inserted into the center comes out clean. Just remember to let all other dog owners know that it contains CBD (and how much) before feeding it to their pups.

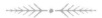

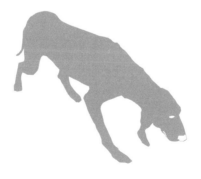

THE ELVIS PUPSLEYS
{ PEANUT BUTTER & BANANA, BABY! }

1 c. bananas
2 c. oat flour
1 tsp. baking powder
¹/₂ tsp. baking soda
³/₄ c. carob chips (do NOT substitute with chocolate)
2 eggs
1 c. peanut butter
1 tsp. vanilla
1 tbsp. honey
¹/₄ c. safflower oil
CBD oil (see page 16 for dosage amounts)

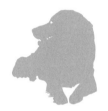

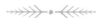

Preheat oven to 350°F. Peel and mash bananas, and then puree in a food processor.

Combine all ingredients together and mix thoroughly. Place cupcake papers into a mini muffin pan. Spoon the mixture evenly into the papers, coming close to the top of the papers (the mix will not rise very much).

Bake 10 to 15 minutes or until a toothpick inserted into the center comes out clean. Transfer and let cool completely on a wire rack. Store in an airtight container in the refrigerator. For more options, read the "Storage Tips" section on page 19.

Note: These can be iced with one of the icing recipes described earlier; the King wouldn't have them any other way. And we're pretty sure that the King also would have wanted toppings on his pupsleys, so here are a few recommendations:

- *Banana slices*

- *Bacon crumbles*

- *Ground peanuts*

- *Strawberry*

Use your imagination, but just stay clear of the toxic items for dogs.

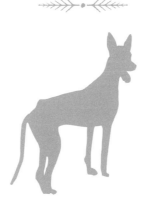

THIS BROWNIE TAKES THE (CHEESE)CAKE

{ TWO GREAT TASTES THAT TASTE GREAT TOGETHER }

....

2 c. oat flour

1 tsp. baking powder

5 tbsp. carob powder (do NOT substitute with chocolate)

1 c. carob chips (do NOT substitute with chocolate)

2 eggs

8-oz. package nonfat cream cheese

¼ c. honey

1 tsp. vanilla

¼ c. safflower oil

CBD oil (see page 16 for dosage amounts)

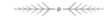

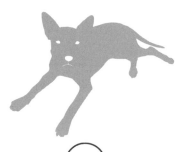

Preheat oven to 325°F. Combine all ingredients together and mix thoroughly. Lightly grease a 9" square baking pan and pour the mixture into it.

Bake for 30 to 35 minutes or until sides loosen from the pan slightly. Transfer and let cool completely on a wire rack. Once cool, slice into individual-sized portions. Store in an airtight container in the refrigerator. For more options, read the "Storage Tips" section on page 19.

Note: These can be iced with one of the icing recipes described earlier.

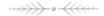

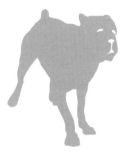

{ CHAPTER 6 }

SOOTHING
Snacks for the
Sensitive
Special treats that meet their needs

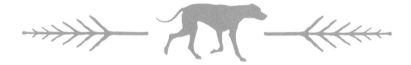

Wouldn't it be nice if we could all eat exactly what we wanted, any time we wanted it? Our bodies, however, aren't built to take that kind of abuse—and neither are those of our dogs. Add to that individual problems like allergies, sensitive stomachs, and so on, and it can sometimes seem like finding anything for them to eat is a chore. This collection of treats is designed to soothe your companion, body and mind, while providing flavor and variety.

Choose to use organic ingredients in these recipes, like we do!

VEGGIE CORNUCOPIA

{ A BOUNTY OF EARTHLY DELIGHTS }

1 ½ c. carrots

½ c. broccoli

½ c. tightly packed spinach leaves

½ c. oat flour

1 ½ c. brown rice flour

½ c. rolled oats (the old-fashioned kind, not instant)

½ c. hulled sunflower seeds (unsalted)

1 egg

CBD oil (see page 16 for dosage amounts)

¼ c. water (add slowly)

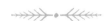

THESE TREATS ARE HIGH IN FIBER, LOW IN FAT, MEAT FREE, AND LOW IN PROTEIN.

Preheat oven to 350°F. Peel and dice carrots, and then finely grind in a food processor. Cook and dice broccoli, and then finely grind in a food processor. Puree spinach in a food processor.

Combine all ingredients (except the water) together. Add water slowly and mix until a dough forms (if too dry, add more water; too wet, add a bit more flour). You may not need all the water if you reach a good consistency first. Line a cookie sheet with parchment paper (for easy cleanup), and spoon out the mixture with a tablespoon and drop onto sheet (they can be rather close together, as they don't grow much while cooking). These cookies will not rise or flatten, so if you want a flatter cookie, press each one down before baking.

Bake 22 to 27 minutes or until golden brown. Transfer and let cool completely on a wire rack. Store the cookies in an airtight container in the refrigerator. For more options, read the "Storage Tips" section on page 19.

CARROTS FOR BREAKFAST...

And lunch, and dinner. Organic carrots are a wonderful regular addition to your dog's diet. They're naturally sweet, crunchy, and nutritious. Many feed their dogs carrot sticks as snacks—and dogs love them! Carrots are an exceptional source of vitamins A and C, as well as potassium. They are also high in fiber. Carrots supply nutrients necessary for the health of the eyes, immune system, and digestive system.

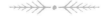

POPEYE POWER PASTRIES

{ ALL I NEEDS IS ME SPINACH }

....

1 c. tightly packed spinach leaves

3 c. garbanzo bean flour (also known as chickpea flour)

$^1/_4$ c. grated Parmesan cheese

1 egg

CBD oil (see page 16 for dosage amounts)

$^1/_2$ c. water (add slowly)

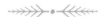

THESE TREATS ARE HIGH IN FIBER, GRAIN FREE AND MEAT FREE.

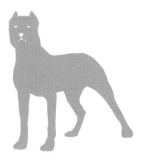

Preheat oven to 350°F. Puree spinach leaves in a food processor until smooth.

Combine all ingredients (except the water) together. Add water slowly and mix until a dough forms (if too dry, add more water; too wet, add a bit more flour). You may not need all the water if you reach a good consistency first. Line a cookie sheet with parchment paper (for easy cleanup), and spoon out the mixture with a tablespoon and drop onto sheet (they can be rather close together, as they don't grow much while cooking). These cookies will not rise or flatten, so if you want a flatter cookie, press each one down before baking.

Bake 22 to 27 minutes or until golden brown. Transfer and let cool completely on a wire rack. Store the cookies in an airtight container in the refrigerator. For more options, read the "Storage Tips" section on page 19.

SPINACH

These treats pack a one-two punch in terms of nutrition and taste. The ingredient combo in these treats is one of the best out there: whole grains, spinach, egg, and cheese. That's energy to burn, and energy to spare. And no shortage of flavor! You may find yourself snacking on these too!

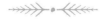

PUMPKIN TO TALK ABOUT

{ GREAT FOR THOSE WITH SENSITIVE TUMMIES }

3 c. garbanzo bean flour (also known as chickpea flour)
$\frac{1}{2}$ c. canned pumpkin (or fresh pureed pumpkin)
1 tsp. cinnamon
1 egg
CBD oil (see page 16 for dosage amounts)
$\frac{1}{3}$ c. water (add slowly)

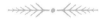

THESE TREATS ARE HIGH IN FIBER, LOW FAT, GRAIN FREE, MEAT FREE, AND LOW PROTEIN .

Preheat oven to 350°F. Combine all ingredients (except the water) together. Add water slowly and mix until a dough forms (if too dry, add more water; too wet, add a bit more flour). You may not need all the water if you reach a good consistency first. Line a cookie sheet with parchment paper (for easy cleanup), and spoon out the mixture with a tablespoon and drop onto sheet (they can be rather close together, as they don't grow much while cooking). These cookies will not rise or flatten, so if you want a flatter cookie, press each one down before baking.

Bake 22 to 27 minutes or until golden brown. Transfer and let cool completely on a wire rack. Store the cookies in an airtight container in the refrigerator. For more options, read the "Storage Tips" section on page 19.

PUMPKIN & YAMS

No, these won't jump out of the cookie jar and fly away, but you will find that your dog loves them so much that you will fly through a batch. Like pumpkins, yams are full of potassium, fiber, beta-carotene, vitamins, and minerals. Mixed with oats and honey, they turn into little "sweet potato pies"—irresistible!

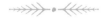

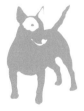

CATCH OF THE DAY

{ GRAIN-FREE FISH TREAT, PERFECT FOR DOGS
THAT SUFFER WITH A LOT OF ALLERGIES }

3 c. tapioca flour (or garbanzo bean flour, or amaranth flour)
2 6-oz. cans wild salmon
1 tsp. dried rosemary
1 tsp. dried parsley
1 tsp. dried oregano
1 tsp. dried sage
CBD oil (see page 16 for dosage amounts)

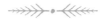

THESE TREATS ARE HIGH PROTEIN, GRAIN FREE, AND FILLED WITH OMEGAS.

Preheat oven to 350°F. Empty entire cans of salmon (juices included) into a food processor and puree.

Combine all ingredients together (if too dry, add water; too wet, add a bit more flour). Line a cookie sheet with parchment paper (for easy cleanup), and spoon out the mixture with a tablespoon and drop onto sheet (they can be rather close together, as they don't grow much while cooking). These cookies will not rise or flatten, so if you want a flatter cookie, press each one down before baking.

Bake 22 to 27 minutes or until golden brown. Transfer and let cool completely on a wire rack. Store the cookies in an airtight container in the refrigerator. For more options, read the "Storage Tips" section on page 19.

SALMON

This delicious, pink-fleshed fish is low in calories and saturated fat, high in protein, and rich in omega-3 fatty acids (the ones that are good for you). Wild-caught, cold-water fish like salmon are higher in omega-3 fatty acids than warm-water fish. Salmon is also an excellent source of selenium, niacin, and vitamin B_{12}, and a good source of phosphorous, magnesium, and vitamin B_6.

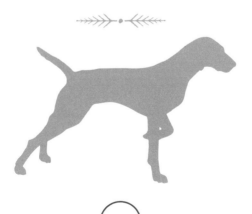

BEEF CHEWS

{ HOMEMADE BEEF JERKY, SAFE AND TASTY! }

1 lb. boneless top round steak or London broil (trimmed of fat)
CBD oil (see page 16 for dosage amounts)

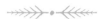

THESE TREATS ARE HIGH PROTEIN
AND GRAIN FREE.

Place beef in a plastic bag with CBD oil and shake to coat. Freeze for 30 to 60 minutes or until firm but not frozen. This allows for easier slicing into thin strips. Use a sharp knife and slice across the grain into thin strips no more than ¼" thick.

Preheat oven to 250°F. Line a cookie sheet with parchment paper (for easy cleanup), and arrange the beef strips in a single layer with a little space between pieces for proper air circulation. Bake for 4 hours, or until dry to the touch. Remove from the oven and let air-dry in a cool place for another 24 hours. Store in an airtight container in the refrigerator. For more options, read the "Storage Tips" section on page 19.

Yields approximately ¾ lb. jerky.

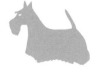

CHICKEN CHEWS

{ HOMEMADE CHICKEN JERKY, SAFE AND TASTY! }

1 lb. boneless, skinless chicken breast (trimmed of fat)
CBD oil (see page 16 for dosage amounts)

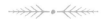

THESE TREATS ARE HIGH PROTEIN
AND GRAIN FREE.

Place chicken in a plastic bag with CBD oil and shake to coat. Freeze for 30 minutes or until firm but not frozen. This allows for easier slicing into thin strips. Use a sharp knife and slice across the grain into thin strips no more than ¼" thick.

Preheat oven to 250°F. Line a cookie sheet with parchment paper (for easy cleanup), and arrange the chicken strips in a single layer with a little space between pieces for proper air circulation. Bake for 4 hours, or until dry to the touch. Remove from the oven and let air-dry in a cool place for another 24 hours. Store in an airtight container in the refrigerator. For more options, read the "Storage Tips" section on page 19.

Yields approximately ¾ lb. jerky.

LIVER LET LIVE

{ RELAX WITH A TREAT }

3 c. amaranth flour (or garbanzo bean flour, or tapioca flour)
1 lb. beef livers (or chicken livers)
2 eggs
CBD oil (see page 16 for dosage amounts)

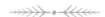

THESE TREATS ARE HIGH PROTEIN
AND GRAIN FREE.

Preheat oven to 300°F. Puree liver in a food processor. Immediately clean it afterward, as liver makes an awful mess if left in there to dry.

Combine all ingredients together and mix thoroughly. Line a jelly roll pan with parchment paper (it helps make cleanup a breeze). Pour the mixture into the pan.

Bake for 30 minutes. Cut into small, individual-sized portions, using a pizza cutter or a knife. Transfer and let cool completely on a wire rack. Store in an airtight container in the refrigerator. For more options, read the "Storage Tips" section on page 19.

Note: To make crunchier treats, put them back in the oven (after cutting them) for an additional 2 hours at 150°F.

GRAIN-FREE FLOURS

Even if your dog isn't gluten intolerant (and be thankful if they aren't), health experts advise going without wheat- and grain-based foods occasionally, and it's helpful to know what to substitute. This recipe is completely grain free—and your dog won't notice or care.

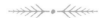

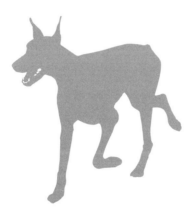

TURKEY JERKY TREAT

{ ONE TOUGH BIRD, BUT ONE
GENTLE-ON-THE-TUMMY TREAT }

1 lb. raw ground turkey (or chicken)
1 tbsp. extra-virgin olive oil
CBD oil (see page 16 for dosage amounts)

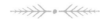

THESE TREATS ARE HIGH PROTEIN,
LOW FAT, AND GRAIN FREE.

Preheat oven to 200°F. Combine all ingredients together in a food processor and puree the mixture. Line a jelly roll pan with parchment paper (it makes cleanup easier) and pour the mixture into it. Spread evenly.

Bake 2 hours with the oven door slightly ajar to allow the moisture to escape. Remove from the oven and, using a pizza cutter or knife, cut into small, individual-sized portions. Place pieces back in the oven, flipped over, and bake an additional 1 to 2 hours or until the treats are dry and leathery. Store in an airtight container in the refrigerator. For more options, read the "Storage Tips" section on page 19.

GOBBLING UP TURKEY

Turkey is a poultry that is becoming more and more available to consumers because it is naturally low in fat without the skin, containing only 1 gram of fat per ounce of flesh. It is also a good source of B vitamins, potassium, and zinc. Cooked with the skin on, the flavor is sealed in without adding fat.

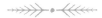

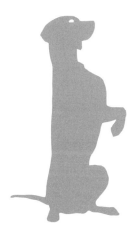

BUFFALO BITES

{ GREAT TO USE AS PURE-MEAT,
HIGH-VALUE TRAINING TREATS }

2 lbs. lean ground beef (or buffalo)
CBD oil (see page 16 for dosage amounts)

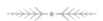

THESE TREATS ARE HIGH PROTEIN, LOW FAT, AND GRAIN FREE.

Preheat oven to 200°F. Puree all ingredients together in a food processor. Line a jelly roll pan with parchment paper (it makes cleanup easier) and pour the mixture into it. Spread evenly.

Bake 2 hours with the oven door slightly ajar to allow the moisture to escape. Remove from the oven and, using a pizza cutter or knife, cut into small, individual-sized portions. Place pieces back in the oven, flipped over, and bake an additional 1 to 2 hours or until the treats are dry and leathery. Store in an airtight container in the refrigerator. For more options, read the "Storage Tips" section on page 19.

HOME ON THE RANGE

Long before settlers moved in and took over, Native Americans were thriving on the multiple blessings of the bison (commonly referred to as the buffalo). One of these was the quality of their meat. In short, bison contains more of what our bodies need—iron, protein, and fatty acids—and less of what we don't (fat, cholesterol, and calories). Because it is nutrient dense, it can be consumed in smaller quantities than beef and still provide similar (if not increased) health benefits while contributing to a greater feeling of fullness. Nutritionally, you get more protein and nutrients with fewer calories and fat than other protein sources. It is also a less common red meat; if your dog has an allergy to beef, they may be quite tolerant of bison.

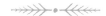

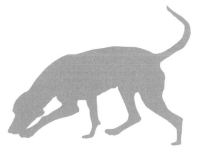

TASTY TUNA TREATS

{ A LOW-FAT, ALLERGY-FRIENDLY TREAT }

1 1/2 c. oat flour
1 1/2 c. brown rice flour
6-oz. can albacore tuna (in water)
1/4 c. oat bran
1 egg
CBD oil (see page 16 for dosage amounts)
1/2 c. water (add slowly)

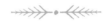

THESE TREATS ARE HIGH PROTEIN,
LOW FAT, ALLERGY FRIENDLY,
AND FILLED WITH BENEFICIAL OMEGAS.

Preheat oven to 350°F. Empty all contents (including juices) from can of tuna into a food processor and puree.

Combine all ingredients (except the water) together. Add water slowly and mix until a dough forms (if too dry, add more water; too wet, add a bit more flour). You may not need all the water if you reach a good consistency first. Roll out on a lightly floured surface to

¼" thickness. Use a cookie cutter (or a knife) to cut into shapes. Line a cookie sheet with parchment paper (for easy cleanup), and place the cookies on the sheet (they can be rather close together, as they don't grow much while cooking).

Bake 22 to 27 minutes or until golden brown. Transfer and let cool completely on a wire rack. Store the cookies in an airtight container in the refrigerator. For more options, read the "Storage Tips" section on page 19.

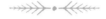

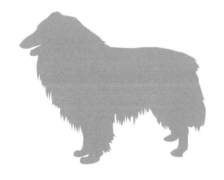

GOING OUT ON A LAMB

{ GRAIN-FREE LAMB TREAT, PERFECT FOR DOGS THAT SUFFER WITH A LOT OF ALLERGIES }

2 c. pumpkin or sweet potato (canned or fresh)
3 c. garbanzo bean flour (or tapioca flour, or amaranth flour)
1 c. ground lamb (precooked and drained)
1 tsp. rosemary
1 tsp. sage
CBD oil (see page 16 for dosage amounts)
½ c. water (add slowly)

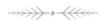

THESE TREATS ARE HIGH PROTEIN, GRAIN FREE, AND ALLERGY FRIENDLY.

Preheat oven to 350°F. If using fresh pumpkin or sweet potato, cook, mash, and puree.

Combine all ingredients (except the water) together. Add water slowly and mix thoroughly (if too dry, add more water; too wet, add a bit more flour). You may not need all the water if you reach a good consistency first. Line a cookie sheet with parchment paper (for easy cleanup), and spoon out the mixture with a tablespoon and drop onto sheet (they can be rather close together, as they don't grow much while cooking). These cookies will not rise or flatten, so if you want a flatter cookie, press each one down before baking.

Bake 22 to 27 minutes or until golden brown. Transfer and let cool completely on a wire rack. Store the cookies in an airtight container in the refrigerator. For more options, read the "Storage Tips" section on page 19.

HERBS FOR LIFE

Whole books have been written on herbs and their health benefits. Sidebars in other chapters of this book have detailed the benefits of some of those most commonly used in dog food (and specifically the treats in this book!). Two particularly interesting websites to visit to learn more include www.crystalgardenherbs.com and www.botanicalmedicine.org.

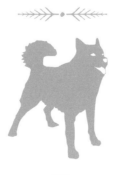

BAD BREATH BEGONE

{ MINTY FRESH }

1 ½ c. oat flour
1 ½ c. brown rice flour
¼ c. applesauce (unsweetened)
½ c. dried mint
½ c. dried parsley
¼ tsp. peppermint oil
1 egg
CBD oil (see page 16 for dosage amounts)
½ c. water (add slowly)

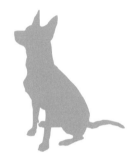

Preheat oven to 350°F. Combine all ingredients (except the water) together. Add water slowly and mix thoroughly (if too dry, add more water; too wet, add a bit more flour). You may not need all the water if you reach a good consistency first. Line a cookie sheet with parchment paper (for easy cleanup), and spoon out the mixture with a tablespoon and drop onto sheet (they can be rather close together, as they don't grow much while cooking). These cookies will not rise or flatten, so if you want a flatter cookie, press each one down before baking. Bake 22 to 27 minutes or until golden brown. Transfer and let cool completely on a wire rack. Store the cookies in an airtight container in the refrigerator. For more options, read the "Storage Tips" section on page 19.

TURKEY BREAST CHEWS

{ HIGH PROTEIN, LOW FAT, GRAIN FREE }

2 lbs. turkey breast (boneless, skinless)
CBD oil (see page 16 for dosage amounts)

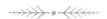

Put turkey in a plastic bag with CBD oil and shake to coat. Place it in the freezer for 30 minutes to allow it to become firmer.

Slice the breast thinly, about ⅛" slices, cutting against the grain (that will make the jerky a little harder to chew and give your dog more time eating it). Try to keep the slices as uniform as possible, so the cook time stays consistent.

Preheat oven to 175°F. Put a wire drying rack on top of a pan, then place the turkey slices on top of the wire rack. Do not overlap the pieces. Bake for 2 hours, then flip the strips and bake another 2 hours. If you want to make the jerky even chewier, cook for additional time, until the desired consistency is reached. Store in an airtight container in the refrigerator. For more options, read the "Storage Tips" section on page 19.

LIVER CHEWS

{ HIGH-VALUE TREAT, GREAT FOR TRAINING }

2 lbs. chicken livers
CBD oil (see page 16 for dosage amounts)

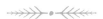

Put chicken livers in a plastic bag with CBD oil and shake to coat. Place in the freezer for 20 minutes to allow them to become firmer. Slice the livers thinly, about ⅛" slices. Try to keep the slices as uniform as possible, so the cook time stays consistent.

Preheat oven to 175°F. Put a wire drying rack on top of a pan, then place the liver slices on top of the wire rack. Do not overlap the pieces. Bake for 2 hours, then flip the strips and bake another 1 to 2 hours. These are smaller, bite-size pieces, so they are great for training. If you want to make larger liver jerky, you can use a beef liver, since it is much bigger. Store in an airtight container in the refrigerator. For more options, read the "Storage Tips" section on page 19.

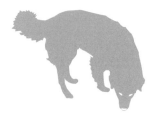

SALMON CHEWS

{ FULL OF OMEGAS, & HEART, SKIN COAT HEALTHY }

2 lbs. salmon fillets (skin-on preferred)
CBD oil (see page 16 for dosage amounts)

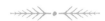

Put salmon in a plastic bag with CBD oil and shake to coat. Place in the freezer for 30 minutes to allow it to become firmer. Slice the fillets thinly, about $1/8$" slices, keeping the skin on. Cut against the grain to make the jerky chewier for your dog. Try to keep the slices as uniform as possible, so the cook time stays consistent.

Preheat oven to 175°F. Put a wire drying rack on top of a pan, then place the salmon slices on top of the wire rack. Do not overlap the pieces. Bake for 2 hours, then flip the strips and bake another 2 hours. These are smaller, bite-size pieces, so they are great for training. Store in an airtight container in the refrigerator. For more options, read the "Storage Tips" section on page 19.

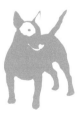

SWEET POTATO JERKY

{ LOW PROTEIN, HIGH FIBER, GREAT FOR SENSITIVE BELLIES }

2 sweet potatoes
CBD oil (see page 16 for dosage amounts)

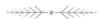

For smaller dogs, slice the sweet potato in rounds, about ¼" thick, keeping the skin on. For larger dogs, slice them into ¼" strips, lengthwise. Try to keep the slices as uniform as possible, so the cook time stays consistent. Put the slices into a plastic bag with CBD oil and shake to coat.

Preheat oven to 250°F. Place slices on a baking sheet lined with parchment. Do not overlap the pieces. Bake for 1.5 hours, then flip the pieces and bake another 1 to 1.5 hours. The longer they stay in the oven, the crispier they'll get; the shorter they stay in, the chewier they'll be. Store in an airtight container in the refrigerator. For more options, read the "Storage Tips" section on page 19.

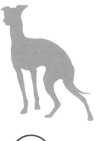

PIG SKIN CHEWS

{ YOUR DOG WILL GO CRAZY FOR THESE! }

2 lbs. pig skin
CBD oil (see page 16 for dosage amounts)

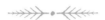

You can buy sliced pig skin in most supermarkets' meat section, and it makes a great treat for your dogs, one that is sure to become a favorite. Slice the skin into evenly sized strips, keeping in mind the size of your dog (we recommend 2" x 6" for medium- to larger-sized dogs, and smaller for smaller dogs). Try to keep the slices as uniform as possible, so the cook time stays consistent. Put the slices into a plastic bag with CBD oil and shake to coat.

Preheat oven to 175°F. Put a wire drying rack on top of a pan, then place the strips on top of the wire rack. Do not overlap the pieces. Bake for 5 hours, then flip the strips and bake another 5 hours. The time will vary depending upon how thick the skins were cut, how much fat was on them, and how crunchy you want them to be. We recommend trying to make them pretty crunchy, but still a bit chewy for a longer-lasting treat. Store in an airtight container in the refrigerator. For more options, read the "Storage Tips" section on page 19.

DRIED APPLE JERKY

{ LOW-FAT, LOW-PROTEIN, HIGH-FIBER SNACKS }

3 apples (Gala, Fuji, Honeycrisp, or Granny Smith)
CBD oil (see page 16 for dosage amounts)

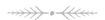

Remove the core and seeds (apple seeds can be toxic to dogs), then slice the apples into ¼" rounds. Try to keep the slices as uniform as possible, so the cook time stays consistent. Put the slices into a plastic bag with CBD oil and shake to coat.

Preheat oven to 200°F. Place slices on a baking sheet lined with parchment. Do not overlap the pieces. Bake for 1.5 hours, then flip the pieces and bake another 1 hour. The longer they stay in the oven, the crispier they'll get; the shorter they stay in, the chewier they'll be. Store in an airtight container in the refrigerator. For more options, read the "Storage Tips" section on page 19.

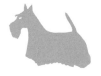

LAMB CHEWS

{ HIGH PROTEIN, LOW FAT, GRAIN FREE, AND AN
ALTERNATIVE PROTEIN SOURCE }

2 lbs. lamb loin or fillet
CBD oil (see page 16 for dosage amounts)

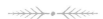

Put lamb in the freezer for 30 minutes to allow it to become firmer. Slice the loin thinly, about $^1/_8$" slices, cutting against the grain. Try to keep the slices as uniform as possible, so the cook time stays consistent. Put the slices into a plastic bag with CBD oil and shake to coat.

Preheat oven to 175°F. Put a wire drying rack on top of a pan, then place the lamb slices on top of the wire rack. Do not overlap the pieces. Bake for 2 hours, then flip the strips and bake another 2 hours. If you want to make the jerky even chewier, cook for additional time, until the desired consistency is reached. Store in an airtight container in the refrigerator. For more options, read the "Storage Tips" section on page 19.

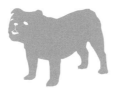

KALE 'EM WITH KINDNESS

{ LOW-FAT, HIGH-FIBER KALE CHIPS
THAT DOGS WILL LOVE }

1 bag or bunch fresh kale
2 tbsp. coconut oil
CBD oil (see page 16 for dosage amounts)

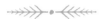

Wash kale, then tear the leaves into bite-size pieces and place in a large mixing bowl. Toss with the coconut oil and CBD oil to evenly coat.

Preheat oven to 350°F. Place leaves on a baking sheet lined with parchment. Do not overlap the pieces. Bake for 12 to 16 minutes. The leaves should still be dark green and not burnt or brown. Let cool completely. Store in an airtight container in the refrigerator. For more options, read the "Storage Tips" section on page 19.

FUN WITH FRUIT LEATHER

{ HIGH FIBER, LOW FAT,
GREAT FOR SENSITIVE TUMMIES }

1 c. applesauce (unsweetened)
2 c. strawberries (fresh or frozen)
CBD oil (see page 16 for dosage amounts)

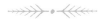

Place all ingredients in a blender or food processor and puree.

Preheat oven to 175°F. Line a baking sheet with parchment paper and then spread the mixture out evenly in the pan, using a spatula. Bake for 6 hours, then remove from the oven and leave the pan on the counter to cool an additional 4 hours (or overnight). Use kitchen scissors to cut the fruit leather into strips (you can leave the parchment paper on at this time and remove it later when you go to feed the treats to your dog). Store in an airtight container in the refrigerator. For more options, read the "Storage Tips" section on page 19.

CHAPTER 7

TRANQUIL
VEGGIE TREATS

High fiber & low protein

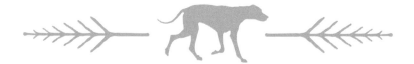

Now, we know dogs love meat, but they also love fruits and veggies. There are a lot of reasons why, as an owner, you would choose to feed your dog a vegetarian or vegan treat—just as there are a lot of reasons why you would choose to give your dog CBD. Maybe it aligns with your own lifestyle choices. Maybe they're overweight or they need more fiber in their diet to regulate their stool. No matter your reasons, these recipes will help your puppy pal be healthy and happy-go-lucky.

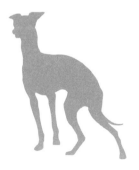

I YAM WHAT I YAM

{ HIGH FIBER, LOW PROTEIN, GREAT FOR SENSITIVE TUMMIES & DIGESTIVE HEALTH }

1 ½ c. oat flour
1 ½ c. brown rice flour
½ c. pureed sweet potato (canned or fresh)
1 large, ripe banana (mashed)
½ tsp. ground cinnamon
CBD oil (see page 16 for dosage amounts)
⅓ c. water (add slowly)

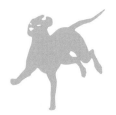

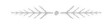

Preheat oven to 350°F. Combine all ingredients (except the water) together. Add water slowly and mix until a dough forms (if too dry, add more water; too wet, add a bit more flour). You may not need all the water to reach the desired consistency. Roll out on a lightly floured surface to ¼" thickness. Use a cookie cutter (or a knife) to cut into shapes. Line a cookie sheet with parchment paper (for easy cleanup) and place the cookies on the sheet (they can be rather close together, as they don't grow much while cooking).

Bake 18 to 25 minutes or until golden brown. Transfer and let cool completely on a wire rack. Store the cookies in an airtight container in the refrigerator. For more options, read the "Storage Tips" section on page 19.

APPLE OF MY EYE

{ ANTIOXIDANT RICH & HIGH IN FIBER }

1 ½ c. oat flour

1 ½ c. brown rice flour

½ c. almond butter (unsalted, natural is best)

½ c. pureed raspberries (frozen or fresh)

½ c. applesauce (unsweetened)

CBD oil (see page 16 for dosage amounts)

⅓ c. water (add slowly)

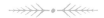

Preheat oven to 350°F. Combine all ingredients (except the water) together. Add water slowly and mix until a dough forms (if too dry, add more water; too wet, add a bit more flour). You may not need all the water to reach the desired consistency. Roll out on a lightly floured surface to ¼" thickness. Use a cookie cutter (or a knife) to cut into shapes. Line a cookie sheet with parchment paper (for easy cleanup) and place the cookies on the sheet (they can be rather close together, as they don't grow much while cooking).

Bake 22 to 30 minutes or until golden brown. Transfer and let cool completely on a wire rack. Store the cookies in an airtight container in the refrigerator. For more options, read the "Storage Tips" section on page 19.

SUNSHINE SNACKS

{ HIGH FIBER, LOW PROTEIN
& FULL OF NUTRIENTS }

1 ½ c. oat flour
1 ½ c. brown rice flour
½ c. pureed strawberries (fresh or frozen)
1 large, ripe banana (mashed)
1 tbsp. honey
CBD oil (see page 16 for dosage amounts)
⅓ c. water (add slowly)

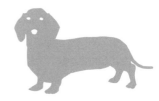

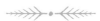

Preheat oven to 350°F. Combine all ingredients (except the water) together. Add water slowly and mix until a dough forms (if too dry, add more water; too wet, add a bit more flour). You may not need all the water to reach the desired consistency. Roll out on a lightly floured surface to ¼" thickness. Use a cookie cutter (or a knife) to cut into shapes. Line a cookie sheet with parchment paper (for easy cleanup) and place the cookies on the sheet (they can be rather close together, as they don't grow much while cooking).

Bake 18 to 25 minutes or until golden brown. Transfer and let cool completely on a wire rack. Store the cookies in an airtight container in the refrigerator. For more options, read the "Storage Tips" section on page 19.

PLEASING PUMPKIN PASTRIES

{ HIGH FIBER & GREAT FOR DIGESTIVE HEALTH }

1 ½ c. oat flour

1 ½ c. brown rice flour

½ c. peanut butter (unsalted, natural is best)

½ c. pureed pumpkin (canned or fresh)

CBD oil (see page 16 for dosage amounts)

½ c. water (add slowly)

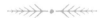

Preheat oven to 350°F. Combine all ingredients (except the water) together. Add water slowly and mix until a dough forms (if too dry, add more water; too wet, add a bit more flour). You may not need all the water to reach the desired consistency. Roll out on a lightly floured surface to ¼" thickness. Use a cookie cutter (or a knife) to cut into shapes. Line a cookie sheet with parchment paper (for easy cleanup) and place the cookies on the sheet (they can be rather close together, as they don't grow much while cooking).

Bake 22 to 30 minutes or until golden brown. Transfer and let cool completely on a wire rack. Store the cookies in an airtight container in the refrigerator. For more options, read the "Storage Tips" section on page 19.

OAT OF THIS WORLD

{ HIGH FIBER, LOW PROTEIN & ANTIOXIDANT RICH }

1 ½ c. oat flour
1 ½ c. brown rice flour
½ c. pureed blueberries (fresh or frozen)
1 large, ripe banana (mashed)
½ c. rolled oats (the old-fashioned kind, not instant)
2 tbsp. flaxseeds
2 tbsp. coconut oil
CBD oil (see page 16 for dosage amounts)
½ c. water (add slowly)

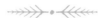

Preheat oven to 350°F. Combine all ingredients (except the water) together. Add water slowly and mix until a dough forms (if too dry, add more water; too wet, add a bit more flour). You may not need all the water to reach the desired consistency. Roll out on a lightly floured surface to ¼" thickness. Use a cookie cutter (or a knife) to cut into shapes. Line a cookie sheet with parchment paper (for easy cleanup) and place the cookies on the sheet (they can be rather close together, as they don't grow much while cooking).

Bake 18 to 25 minutes or until golden brown. Transfer and let cool completely on a wire rack. Store the cookies in an airtight container in the refrigerator. For more options, read the "Storage Tips" section on page 19.

GO COCO-NUTS

{ HIGH FIBER, LOW PROTEIN & GREAT FOR SKIN, COAT & INFLAMMATION ISSUES }

1 ½ c. oat flour
1 ½ c. brown rice flour
1 c. tightly packed kale leaves (pureed)
½ tsp. ground turmeric
¼ c. coconut oil
CBD oil (see page 16 for dosage amounts)
¼ c. water (add slowly)

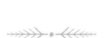

Preheat oven to 350°F. Combine all ingredients (except the water) together. Add water slowly and mix until a dough forms (if too dry, add more water; too wet, add a bit more flour). You may not need all the water to reach the desired consistency. Roll out on a lightly floured surface to ¼" thickness. Use a cookie cutter (or a knife) to cut into shapes. Line a cookie sheet with parchment paper (for easy cleanup) and place the cookies on the sheet (they can be rather close together, as they don't grow much while cooking).

Bake 18 to 25 minutes or until golden brown. Transfer and let cool completely on a wire rack. Store the cookies in an airtight container in the refrigerator. For more options, read the "Storage Tips" section on page 19.

KEEP CALM & CARROT ON

{ HIGH FIBER, LOW PROTEIN & FULL OF VITAMINS }

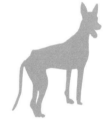

1 ½ c. oat flour

1 ½ c. brown rice flour

½ c. pureed pumpkin (canned or fresh)

½ c. pureed carrots

½ c. applesauce (unsweetened)

CBD oil (see page 16 for dosage amounts)

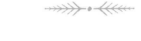

Preheat oven to 350°F. Combine all ingredients together. If too dry, add 1 tablespoon of water at a time to reach desired consistency. If it gets too wet, add more flour. Roll out on a lightly floured surface to ¼" thickness. Use a cookie cutter (or a knife) to cut into shapes. Line a cookie sheet with parchment paper (for easy cleanup) and place the cookies on the sheet (they can be rather close together, as they don't grow much while cooking).

Bake 18 to 25 minutes or until golden brown. Transfer and let cool completely on a wire rack. Store the cookies in an airtight container in the refrigerator. For more options, read the "Storage Tips" section on page 19.

YES I CRAN-BERRY

{ ANTIOXIDANT RICH, LOW PROTEIN & GREAT FOR
SKIN, COAT & KIDNEY HEALTH }

1 ½ c. oat flour
1 ½ c. brown rice flour
½ c. dried cranberries
½ c. shredded coconut (unsweetened)
1 large, ripe banana (mashed)
2 tbsp. coconut oil
CBD oil (see page 16 for dosage amounts)
½ c. coconut water (add slowly)

Preheat oven to 350°F. Combine all ingredients (except the coconut water) together. Add coconut water slowly and mix until a dough forms (if too dry, add more coconut water; too wet, add a bit more flour). You may not need all the coconut water to reach the desired consistency. Roll out on a lightly floured surface to ¼" thickness. Use a cookie cutter (or a knife) to cut into shapes. Line a cookie sheet with parchment paper (for easy cleanup) and place the cookies on the sheet (they can be rather close together, as they don't grow much while cooking).

Bake 18 to 25 minutes or until golden brown. Transfer and let cool completely on a wire rack. Store the cookies in an airtight container in the refrigerator. For more options, read the "Storage Tips" section on page 19.

EVERYTHING IS GONNA BE O-KALE

{ HIGH FIBER, LOW PROTEIN & GREAT FOR SKIN, COAT & SENSITIVE BELLIES }

1 $\frac{1}{2}$ c. oat flour
1 $\frac{1}{2}$ c. brown rice flour
1 c. tightly packed kale leaves (pureed)
1 c. pureed sweet potato (fresh or canned)
2 tbsp. flax seeds
$\frac{1}{4}$ c. coconut oil
CBD oil (see page 16 for dosage amounts)
$\frac{1}{4}$ c. water (add slowly)

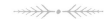

Preheat oven to 350°F. Combine all ingredients (except the water) together. Add water slowly and mix until a dough forms (if too dry, add more water; too wet, add a bit more flour). You may not need all the water to reach the desired consistency. Roll out on a lightly floured surface to $\frac{1}{4}$" thickness. Use a cookie cutter (or a knife) to cut into shapes. Line a cookie sheet with parchment paper (for easy cleanup) and place the cookies on the sheet (they can be rather close together, as they don't grow much while cooking).

Bake 18 to 25 minutes or until golden brown. Transfer and let cool completely on a wire rack. Store the cookies in an airtight container in the refrigerator. For more options, read the "Storage Tips" section on page 19.

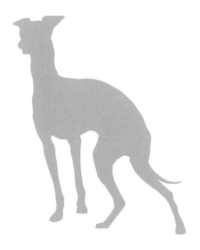

P.B., BERRY & BANANA COOKIES

{ ANTIOXIDANT RICH, FULL OF VITAMINS & A TASTE DOGS LOVE }

1 ½ c. oat flour

1 ½ c. brown rice flour

½ c. pureed blueberries (fresh or frozen)

½ c. peanut butter (unsalted)

1 large, ripe banana (mashed)

1 tbsp. honey

½ tsp. ground cinnamon

CBD oil (see page 16 for dosage amounts)

⅓ c. water (add slowly)

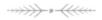

Preheat oven to 350°F. Combine all ingredients (except the water) together. Add water slowly and mix until a dough forms (if too dry, add more water; too wet, add a bit more flour). You may not need all the water to reach the desired consistency. Roll out on a lightly floured surface to ¼" thickness. Use a cookie cutter (or a knife) to cut into shapes. Line a cookie sheet with parchment paper (for easy cleanup) and place the cookies on the sheet (they can be rather close together, as they don't grow much while cooking).

Bake 18 to 25 minutes or until golden brown. Transfer and let cool completely on a wire rack. Store the cookies in an airtight container in the refrigerator. For more options, read the "Storage Tips" section on page 19.

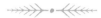

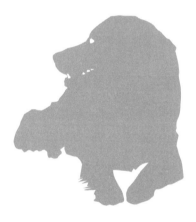

CHAPTER 8

QUICK&

Calming Cookies

Simple & easy

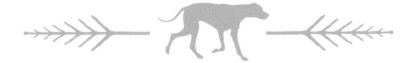

We know you're busy. Who isn't?! Life can be overwhelming and exhausting. For your dog too—even if they're mostly busy sleeping and chasing their tail. That's why we created this chapter, filled with 20 simple recipes with minimal ingredients (many of which you likely already have in your kitchen), along with calming, healing CBD. Your dog's going to be drooling at the smell of them.

BEST OF BROTH WORLDS

{ BONE BROTH & TURMERIC—NUTRIENT DENSE, EASY & HEALTHY }

1 ½ c. oat flour
1 ½ c. brown rice flour
1 tsp. ground turmeric
1 egg
CBD oil (see page 16 for dosage amounts)
½ c. bone broth (add slowly)

Preheat oven to 350°F. Combine all ingredients (except the broth) together. Add broth slowly and mix until a dough forms (if too dry, add more broth; too wet, add a bit more flour). You may not need all of the broth to reach the desired consistency. Roll out on a lightly floured surface to ¼" thickness. Use a cookie cutter (or a knife) to cut into shapes. Line a cookie sheet with parchment paper (for easy cleanup) and place the cookies on the sheet (they can be rather close together, as they don't grow much while cooking).

Bake 22 to 27 minutes or until golden brown. Transfer and let cool completely on a wire rack. Store the cookies in an airtight container in the refrigerator. For more options, read the "Storage Tips" section on page 19.

Note: We recommend using beef bone broth (you can make it yourself with your leftover bones or ones you buy from the butcher, or you can purchase premade bone broth). You can also use poultry, pork, bison, or lamb broth for these tasty biscuits.

NUTS ABOUT BANANAS

{ SO TASTY, YOU'RE GONNA WANT SOME TOO }

1 ½ c. oat flour
1 ½ c. brown rice flour
½ c. peanut butter
1 large banana (extra ripe, mashed)
CBD oil (see page 16 for dosage amounts)
½ c. water (add slowly)

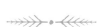

Preheat oven to 350°F. Combine all ingredients (except the water) together. Add water slowly and mix until a dough forms (if too dry, add more water; too wet, add a bit more flour). You may not need all the water to reach the desired consistency. Roll out on a lightly floured surface to ¼" thickness. Use a cookie cutter (or a knife) to cut the dough into the desired shapes. Line a cookie sheet with parchment paper (for easy cleanup) and place the cookies on the sheet (they can be rather close together, as they don't grow much while cooking).

Bake 22 to 30 minutes or until golden brown. Transfer and let cool completely on a wire rack. Store the cookies in an airtight container in the refrigerator. For more options, read the "Storage Tips" section on page 19.

BASIL CHICKEN

{ PROTEIN RICH, ANTIVIRAL
& SMELLS GREAT }

1 ½ c. oat flour
1 ½ c. brown rice flour
½ c. ground chicken (precooked)
1 tbsp. ground basil
1 egg
CBD oil (see page 16 for dosage amounts)
½ c. water (add slowly)

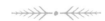

Preheat oven to 350°F. Combine all ingredients (except the water) together. Add water slowly and mix until a dough forms (if too dry, add more water; too wet, add a bit more flour). You may not need all the water to reach the desired consistency. Roll out on a lightly floured surface to ¼" thickness. Use a cookie cutter (or a knife) to cut the dough into the desired shapes. Line a cookie sheet with parchment paper (for easy cleanup) and place the cookies on the sheet (they can be rather close together, as they don't grow much while cooking).

Bake 22 to 27 minutes or until golden brown. Transfer and let cool completely on a wire rack. Store the cookies in an airtight container in the refrigerator. For more options, read the "Storage Tips" section on page 19.

DON'T BE BLUE(BERRY)

{ ANTIOXIDANT RICH, TASTY & VEGETARIAN }

1 ½ c. oat flour

1 ½ c. brown rice flour

½ c. almond butter (unsalted, natural is best)

½ c. pureed blueberries (frozen or fresh)

CBD oil (see page 16 for dosage amounts)

½ c. water (add slowly)

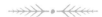

Preheat oven to 350°F. Combine all ingredients (except the water) together. Add water slowly and mix until a dough forms (if too dry, add more water; too wet, add a bit more flour). You may not need all the water to reach the desired consistency. Roll out on a lightly floured surface to ¼" thickness. Use a cookie cutter (or a knife) to cut the dough into the desired shapes. Line a cookie sheet with parchment paper (for easy cleanup) and place the cookies on the sheet (they can be rather close together, as they don't grow much while cooking).

Bake 22 to 30 minutes or until golden brown. Transfer and let cool completely on a wire rack. Store the cookies in an airtight container in the refrigerator. For more options, read the "Storage Tips" section on page 19.

THE TUR-KEY TO SUCCESS

{ LOW FAT, HIGH FIBER & SUPER TASTY }

1 ½ c. oat flour

1 ½ c. brown rice flour

½ c. ground turkey (precooked)

½ c. pureed carrots

1 egg

CBD oil (see page 16 for dosage amounts)

½ c. water (add slowly)

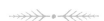

Preheat oven to 350°F. Combine all ingredients (except the water) together. Add water slowly and mix until a dough forms (if too dry, add more water; too wet, add a bit more flour). You may not need all the water to reach the desired consistency. Roll out on a lightly floured surface to ¼" thickness. Use a cookie cutter (or a knife) to cut the dough into the desired shapes. Line a cookie sheet with parchment paper (for easy cleanup) and place the cookies on the sheet (they can be rather close together, as they don't grow much while cooking).

Bake 22 to 27 minutes or until golden brown. Transfer and let cool completely on a wire rack. Store the cookies in an airtight container in the refrigerator. For more options, read the "Storage Tips" section on page 19.

HONEY, I'M HOME

{ TREATS FOR WHEN YOU COME HOME TO
YOUR BFF, HIGH IN FIBER & GREAT FOR
SENSITIVE TUMMIES }

1 ½ c. oat flour
1 ½ c. brown rice flour
½ c. pureed pumpkin (canned or fresh)
1 tbsp. honey
CBD oil (see page 16 for dosage amounts)
½ c. water (add slowly)

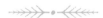

Preheat oven to 350°F. Combine all ingredients (except the water) together. Add water slowly and mix until a dough forms (if too dry, add more water; too wet, add a bit more flour). You may not need all the water to reach the desired consistency. Roll out on a lightly floured surface to ¼" thickness. Use a cookie cutter (or a knife) to cut the dough into the desired shapes. Line a cookie sheet with parchment paper (for easy cleanup), and place the cookies on the sheet (they can be rather close together, as they don't grow much while cooking).

Bake 22 to 30 minutes or until golden brown. Transfer and let cool completely on a wire rack. Store the cookies in an airtight container in the refrigerator. For more options, read the "Storage Tips" section on page 19.

LET'S BEEF FRIENDS

{ RICH IN PROTEIN & BREATH FRESHENING }

1 ½ c. oat flour
1 ½ c. brown rice flour
½ c. ground beef (precooked)
2 tbsp. ground parsley
1 egg
CBD oil (see page 16 for dosage amounts)
½ c. water (add slowly)

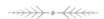

Preheat oven to 350°F. Combine all ingredients (except the water) together. Add water slowly and mix until a dough forms (if too dry, add more water; too wet, add a bit more flour). You may not need all the water to reach the desired consistency. Roll out on a lightly floured surface to ¼" thickness. Use a cookie cutter (or a knife) to cut the dough into the desired shapes. Line a cookie sheet with parchment paper (for easy cleanup), and place the cookies on the sheet (they can be rather close together, as they don't grow much while cooking).

Bake 22 to 27 minutes or until golden brown. Transfer and let cool completely on a wire rack. Store the cookies in an airtight container in the refrigerator. For more options, read the "Storage Tips" section on page 19.

CINNA-YUM COOKIES

{ FULL OF VITAMINS, LOW PROTEIN & GREAT FOR
KIDNEY OR LIVER AILMENTS }

1 1/2 c. oat flour
1 1/2 c. brown rice flour
1/2 c. applesauce (unsweetened)
1 tsp. ground cinnamon
CBD oil (see page 16 for dosage amounts)
1/2 c. water (add slowly)

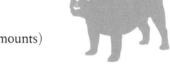

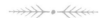

Preheat oven to 350°F. Combine all ingredients (except the water) together. Add water slowly and mix until a dough forms (if too dry, add more water; too wet, add a bit more flour). You may not need all the water to reach the desired consistency. Roll out on a lightly floured surface to 1/4" thickness. Use a cookie cutter (or a knife) to cut the dough into the desired shapes. Line a cookie sheet with parchment paper (for easy cleanup) and place the cookies on the sheet (they can be rather close together, as they don't grow much while cooking).

Bake 22 to 30 minutes or until golden brown. Transfer and let cool completely on a wire rack. Store the cookies in an airtight container in the refrigerator. For more options, read the "Storage Tips" section on page 19.

SWEET POTATO SALMON

{ OMEGA RICH & GREAT FOR SKIN, COAT & HEART HEALTH }

1 ½ c. oat flour

1 ½ c. brown rice flour

6-oz. can wild-caught salmon

½ c. pureed sweet potato (canned or fresh)

1 egg

CBD oil (see page 16 for dosage amounts)

½ c. water (add slowly)

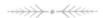

Preheat oven to 350°F. Combine all ingredients (except the water) together, and use all the liquid from the can of salmon; dogs love that! Add water slowly and mix until a dough forms (if too dry, add more water; too wet, add a bit more flour). You may not need all the water to reach the desired consistency. Roll out on a lightly floured surface to ¼" thickness. Use a cookie cutter (or a knife) to cut the dough into the desired shapes. Line a cookie sheet with parchment paper (for easy cleanup), and place the cookies on the sheet (they can be rather close together, as they don't grow much while cooking).

Bake 22 to 27 minutes or until golden brown. Transfer and let cool completely on a wire rack. Store the cookies in an airtight container in the refrigerator. For more options, read the "Storage Tips" section on page 19.

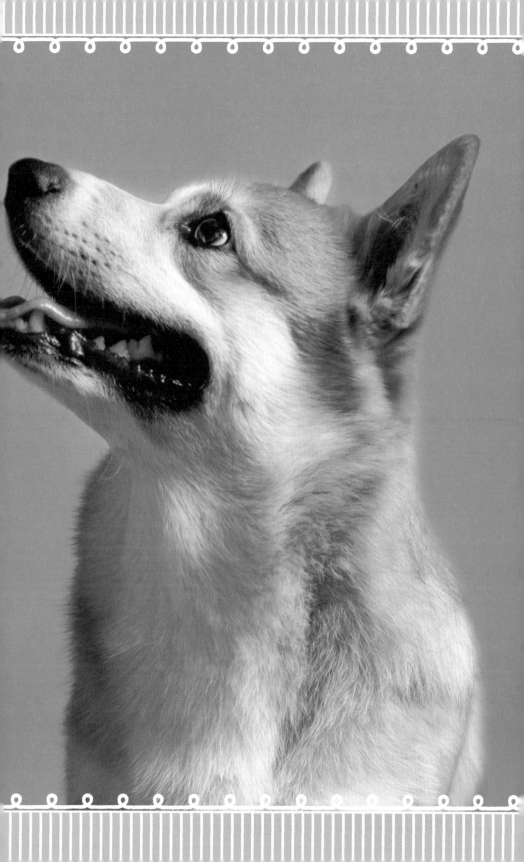

WHAT'S SHAKIN', BACON

{ THESE MIGHT BE DOGS' FAVORITE TWO
INGREDIENTS—THIS WILL BE A GO-TO RECIPE }

1 ½ c. oat flour
1 ½ c. brown rice flour
½ c. peanut butter (unsalted, natural)
6 slices cooked bacon (ground)
CBD oil (see page 16 for dosage amounts)
½ c. water (add slowly)

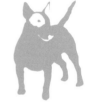

→→→》•《←←←

Preheat oven to 350°F. Combine all ingredients (except the water) together. Add water slowly and mix until a dough forms (if too dry, add more water; too wet, add a bit more flour). You may not need all the water to reach the desired consistency. Roll out on a lightly floured surface to ¼" thickness. Use a cookie cutter (or a knife) to cut the dough into the desired shapes. Line a cookie sheet with parchment paper (for easy cleanup) and place the cookies on the sheet (they can be rather close together, as they don't grow much while cooking).

Bake 22 to 30 minutes or until golden brown. Transfer and let cool completely on a wire rack. Store the cookies in an airtight container in the refrigerator. For more options, read the "Storage Tips" section on page 19.

LOTSA MOZZARELLA

{ COME ON, WHOSE DOG DOESN'T
LOVE PIZZA CRUSTS?! }

1 ½ c. oat flour
1 ½ c. brown rice flour
½ c. shredded low fat mozzarella cheese
1 tbsp. ground oregano
1 egg
CBD oil (see page 16 for dosage amounts)
½ c. water (add slowly)

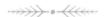

Preheat oven to 350°F. Combine all ingredients (except the water) together. Add water slowly and mix until a dough forms (if too dry, add more water; too wet, add a bit more flour). You may not need all the water to reach the desired consistency. Roll out on a lightly floured surface to ¼" thickness. Use a cookie cutter (or a knife) to cut the dough into the desired shapes. Line a cookie sheet with parchment paper (for easy cleanup) and place the cookies on the sheet (they can be rather close together, as they don't grow much while cooking).

Bake 22 to 27 minutes or until golden brown. Transfer and let cool completely on a wire rack. Store the cookies in an airtight container in the refrigerator. For more options, read the "Storage Tips" section on page 19.

PUMPKIN CRANBERRY COOKIES

{ HIGH IN FIBER, ANTIOXIDANT RICH & GREAT FOR KIDNEY HEALTH }

1 ½ c. oat flour
1 ½ c. brown rice flour
½ c. pureed pumpkin (canned or fresh)
½ c. dried cranberries (pureed)
CBD oil (see page 16 for dosage amounts)
½ c. water (add slowly)

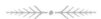

Preheat oven to 350°F. Combine all ingredients (except the water) together. Add water slowly and mix until a dough forms (if too dry, add more water, too wet, add a bit more flour). You may not need all the water to reach the desired consistency. Roll out on a lightly floured surface to ¼" thickness. Use a cookie cutter (or a knife) to cut the dough into the desired shapes. Line a cookie sheet with parchment paper (for easy cleanup) and place the cookies on the sheet (they can be rather close together, as they don't grow much while cooking).

Bake 22 to 30 minutes or until golden brown. Transfer and let cool completely on a wire rack. Store the cookies in an airtight container in the refrigerator. For more options, read the "Storage Tips" section on page 19.

CHILL-FLAX, DAWG

{ HIGH IN PROTEIN, VITAMINS, MINERALS & OMEGAS }

1 ½ c. oat flour
1 ½ c. brown rice flour
½ c. raw beef or chicken liver (pureed)
2 tbsp. flaxseeds
1 egg
CBD oil (see page 16 for dosage amounts)
½ c. water (add slowly)

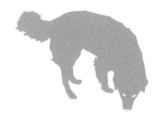

Preheat oven to 350°F. Combine all ingredients (except the water) together. Add water slowly and mix until a dough forms (if too dry, add more water; too wet, add a bit more flour). You may not need all the water to reach the desired consistency. Roll out on a lightly floured surface to ¼" thickness. Use a cookie cutter (or a knife) to cut the dough into the desired shapes. Line a cookie sheet with parchment paper (for easy cleanup) and place the cookies on the sheet (they can be rather close together, as they don't grow much while cooking).

Bake 22 to 27 minutes or until golden brown. Transfer and let cool completely on a wire rack. Store the cookies in an airtight container in the refrigerator. For more options, read the "Storage Tips" section on page 19.

Note: Liver is not the best-smelling meat, so we highly recommend you wash your food processor right after pureeing the liver.

COCO- & PEA-NUT COOKIES

{ GREAT FOR SKIN, COAT & DIGESTIVE HEALTH & OH, SO TASTY }

1 ½ c. oat flour
1 ½ c. brown rice flour
½ c. peanut butter (unsalted, natural)
¼ c. coconut oil
CBD oil (see page 16 for dosage amounts)
¼ c. water (add slowly)

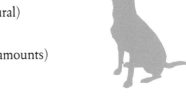

>>>>> • <<<<<

Preheat oven to 350°F. Combine all ingredients (except the water) together. Add water slowly and mix until a dough forms (if too dry, add more water; too wet, add a bit more flour). You may not need all the water to reach the desired consistency. Roll out on a lightly floured surface to ¼" thickness. Use a cookie cutter (or a knife) to cut the dough into the desired shapes. Line a cookie sheet with parchment paper (for easy cleanup) and place the cookies on the sheet (they can be rather close together, as they don't grow much while cooking).

Bake 22 to 30 minutes or until golden brown. Transfer and let cool completely on a wire rack. Store the cookies in an airtight container in the refrigerator. For more options, read the "Storage Tips" section on page 19.

BRING HOME THE BACON

{ THIS IS AN ALL-TIME DOG FAVORITE—
YOU CAN'T GO WRONG HERE }

1 $\frac{1}{2}$ c. oat flour
1 $\frac{1}{2}$ c. brown rice flour
6 slices cooked bacon (ground)
$\frac{1}{2}$ c. shredded low fat cheddar cheese
1 egg
CBD oil (see page 16 for dosage amounts)
$\frac{1}{2}$ c. water (add slowly)

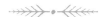

Preheat oven to 350°F. Combine all ingredients (except the water) together. Add water slowly and mix until a dough forms (if too dry, add more water; too wet, add a bit more flour). You may not need all the water to reach the desired consistency. Roll out on a lightly floured surface to $\frac{1}{4}$" thickness. Use a cookie cutter (or a knife) to cut the dough into the desired shapes. Line a cookie sheet with parchment paper (for easy cleanup) and place the cookies on the sheet (they can be rather close together, as they don't grow much while cooking).

Bake 22 to 27 minutes or until golden brown. Transfer and let cool completely on a wire rack. Store the cookies in an airtight container in the refrigerator. For more options, read the "Storage Tips" section on page 19.

FUN ON THE FARM

{ HIGH IN FIBER, POTASSIUM & ANTIOXIDANTS,
LOW IN PROTEIN }

1 ½ c. oat flour

1 ½ c. brown rice flour

½ c. pureed sweet potato (canned or fresh)

½ c. applesauce (unsweetened)

1 egg

CBD oil (see page 16 for dosage amounts)

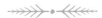

Preheat oven to 350°F. Combine all ingredients together. Mix until a dough forms (if too dry, add 1 tablespoon of water at a time; too wet, add a bit more flour). Roll out on a lightly floured surface to ¼" thickness. Use a cookie cutter (or a knife) to cut the dough into the desired shapes. Line a cookie sheet with parchment paper (for easy cleanup) and place the cookies on the sheet (they can be rather close together, as they don't grow much while cooking).

Bake 22 to 30 minutes or until golden brown. Transfer and let cool completely on a wire rack. Store the cookies in an airtight container in the refrigerator. For more options, read the "Storage Tips" section on page 19.

MINT CONDITION

{ A GREAT ALTERNATIVE PROTEIN SOURCE & BREATH FRESHENING }

1 ½ c. oat flour
1 ½ c. brown rice flour
½ c. ground lamb (precooked)
¼ c. fresh mint leaves (finely chopped)
1 egg
CBD oil (see page 16 for dosage amounts)
½ c. water (add slowly)

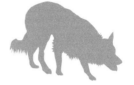

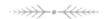

Preheat oven to 350°F. Combine all ingredients (except the water) together. Add water slowly and mix until a dough forms (if too dry, add more water; too wet, add a bit more flour). You may not need all the water to reach the desired consistency. Roll out on a lightly floured surface to ¼" thickness. Use a cookie cutter (or a knife) to cut the dough into the desired shapes. Line a cookie sheet with parchment paper (for easy cleanup) and place the cookies on the sheet (they can be rather close together, as they don't grow much while cooking).

Bake 22 to 27 minutes or until golden brown. Transfer and let cool completely on a wire rack. Store the cookies in an airtight container in the refrigerator. For more options, read the "Storage Tips" section on page 19.

PUMPKIN KALE COOKIES

{ VITAMIN PACKED FOR BONE, HEART & DIGESTIVE HEALTH }

1 c. kale (chopped and tightly packed)
1 ½ c. oat flour
1 ½ c. brown rice flour
½ c. pureed pumpkin (canned or fresh)
CBD oil (see page 16 for dosage amounts)
½ c. water (add slowly)

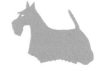

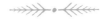

Preheat oven to 350°F. Puree the kale in a food processor. Combine all ingredients (except the water) together. Add water slowly and mix until a dough forms (if too dry, add more water; too wet, add a bit more flour). You may not need all the water to reach the desired consistency. Roll out on a lightly floured surface to ¼" thickness. Use a cookie cutter (or a knife) to cut the dough into the desired shapes. Line a cookie sheet with parchment paper (for easy cleanup) and place the cookies on the sheet (they can be rather close together, as they don't grow much while cooking).

Bake 22 to 30 minutes or until golden brown. Transfer and let cool completely on a wire rack. Store the cookies in an airtight container in the refrigerator. For more options, read the "Storage Tips" section on page 19.

ROSEMARY BISON BITES

{ A HEALTHIER RED MEAT OPTION, EASIER FOR DOGS WITH SENSITIVITIES TO BEEF }

1 ½ c. oat flour
1 ½ c. brown rice flour
½ c. ground bison (precooked)
2 tbsp. dried rosemary (ground)
1 egg
CBD oil (see page 16 for dosage amounts)
½ c. water (add slowly)

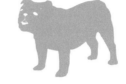

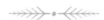

Preheat oven to 350°F. Combine all ingredients (except the water) together. Add water slowly and mix until a dough forms (if too dry, add more water; too wet, add a bit more flour). You may not need all the water to reach the desired consistency. Roll out on a lightly floured surface to ¼" thickness. Use a cookie cutter (or a knife) to cut the dough into the desired shapes. Line a cookie sheet with parchment paper (for easy cleanup) and place the cookies on the sheet (they can be rather close together, as they don't grow much while cooking).

Bake 22 to 27 minutes or until golden brown. Transfer and let cool completely on a wire rack. Store the cookies in an airtight container in the refrigerator. For more options, read the "Storage Tips" section on page 19.

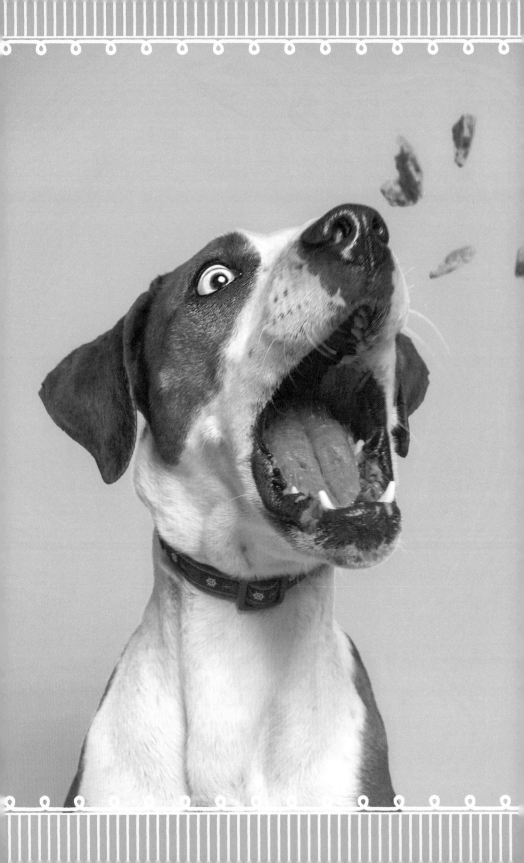

CAROB FOR YOUR CHERUB

{ CAROB IS A HEALTHY ALTERNATIVE TO
CHOCOLATE THAT'S TASTY & SAFE FOR DOGS }

1 ½ c. oat flour

1 ½ c. brown rice flour

½ c. peanut butter (unsalted, natural)

½ c. carob powder (do NOT substitute with chocolate)

1 egg

CBD oil (see page 16 for dosage amounts)

½ c. water (add slowly)

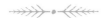

Preheat oven to 350°F. Combine all ingredients (except the water) together. Add water slowly and mix until a dough forms (if too dry, add more water; too wet, add a bit more flour). You may not need all the water to reach the desired consistency. Roll out on a lightly floured surface to ¼" thickness. Use a cookie cutter (or a knife) to cut the dough into the desired shapes. Line a cookie sheet with parchment paper (for easy cleanup) and place the cookies on the sheet (they can be rather close together, as they don't grow much while cooking).

Bake 22 to 30 minutes or until golden brown. Transfer and let cool completely on a wire rack. Store the cookies in an airtight container in the refrigerator. For more options, read the "Storage Tips" section on page 19.

CHAPTER 9

PEACEFUL PUPSICLES

For those warm summer days (& nights)

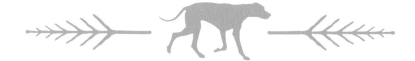

These simple, quick, no-cook treats are the fastest and easiest ways to keep your pup cool—in every sense of the word—on a warm summer day. The best part is that they require no baking—yes, that's right! You just need an ice cube or popsicle tray (small paper cups will also work), and you can make your dog their very own frosty treat, free from preservatives and full of healthy, beneficial ingredients, including CBD.

STRAWBERRY BANANA PUPSICLES

{ COLD, REFRESHING & FULL OF VITAMINS }

1 c. pureed strawberries (fresh or frozen)

1 large banana (mashed and pureed)

1 c. plain nonfat yogurt

1 c. coconut water

CBD oil (see page 16 for dosage amounts)

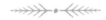

Combine all ingredients together and stir thoroughly. Pour the mixture into an ice cube or popsicle tray. Freeze until solid (at least 4 hours).

CHICKEN GAZPACHO

{ GREAT SAVORY TASTE }

2 ½ c. chicken broth
½ c. carrots (shredded)
½ c. peas (frozen or canned)
1 tsp. ground parsley
CBD oil (see page 16 for dosage amounts)

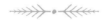

Combine all ingredients together and stir thoroughly. Pour the mixture into an ice cube or popsicle tray. Freeze until solid (at least 4 hours).

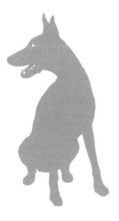

BLUEBERRY OAT PUPSICLES

{ DOGS DESERVE THEIR OWN ANTIOXIDANT-RICH FROZEN YOGURT TREAT }

1 c. blueberries (fresh or frozen)
$\frac{1}{2}$ c. rolled oats (the old-fashioned kind, not instant)
2 c. plain nonfat yogurt
CBD oil (see page 16 for dosage amounts)

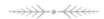

Combine all ingredients together and stir thoroughly. Pour the mixture into an ice cube or popsicle tray. Freeze until solid (at least 4 hours).

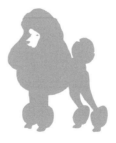

PEANUT BUTTER BACON PUPSICLES

{ ASK YOUR PUP: IS THERE A TASTIER COMBO THAN BACON & PEANUT BUTTER? }

4 slices cooked bacon

½ c. peanut butter (unsalted, natural)

2 c. plain nonfat yogurt

CBD oil (see page 16 for dosage amounts)

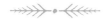

Finely chop the bacon. Combine all ingredients together and stir thoroughly. Pour the mixture into an ice cube or popsicle tray. Freeze until solid (at least 4 hours).

FRESH WATERMELON PUPSICLES

{ PERFECT FOR THAT SUMMER BARBECUE OR DAY AT THE DOG PARK }

2 c. fresh watermelon (cubed)

1 c. coconut water

¼ c. flaxseeds

CBD oil (see page 16 for dosage amounts)

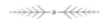

Put all ingredients in a blender and mix until smooth. Pour the mixture into an ice cube or popsicle tray. Freeze until solid (at least 4 hours).

Note: Make these extra special by inserting your dog's favorite biscuit or chew into the wells of the ice cube tray. Then these little doggy ice pops will have everyone wanting seconds.

PEANUT BUTTER BANANA PUPSICLES

{ QUICK, EASY & SURE TO PLEASE ANY DOG }

$^{1}/_{2}$ c. peanut butter (unsalted, natural)

1 ripe medium banana (mashed)

2 c. plain nonfat yogurt

CBD oil (see page 16 for dosage amounts)

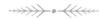

Combine all ingredients together and stir thoroughly. Pour the mixture into an ice cube or popsicle tray. Freeze until solid (at least 4 hours).

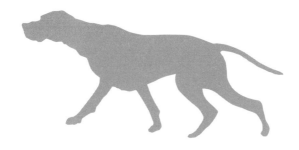

BONE BROTH, TURMERIC & FLAXSEED PUPSICLES

{ A SUPERFOOD DELIGHT FOR YOUR PUP }

2 c. bone broth (beef, pork, or poultry)
½ tsp. turmeric
1 tbsp. flaxseeds
CBD oil (see page 16 for dosage amounts)

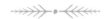

Combine all ingredients together and stir thoroughly. Pour the mixture into an ice cube or popsicle tray. Freeze until solid (at least 4 hours).

Note: Best enjoyed outside, or you can put the treat in their food bowl, so you don't end up with thawed bone broth on your floor.

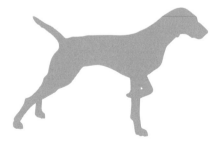

CRANBERRY, ALMOND & COCONUT PUPSICLES

{ REFRESHING & FILLED WITH PROTEIN—
THIS ONE'S A WINNER }

2 c. plain nonfat yogurt

1/2 c. dried cranberries

1/2 c. almond butter (unsalted, natural)

1 c. coconut water

CBD oil (see page 16 for dosage amounts)

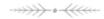

Combine all ingredients together and stir thoroughly. Pour the mixture into an ice cube or popsicle tray. Freeze until solid (at least 4 hours).

BERRY SWEET PUPSICLES

{ CHOCK-FULL OF VITAMINS & ANTIOXIDANTS— THIS IS A CROWD-PLEASER }

½ c. blueberries (fresh or frozen)
½ c. strawberries (finely chopped)
½ c. dried cranberries
2 c. plain nonfat yogurt
CBD oil (see page 16 for dosage amounts)

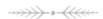

Combine all ingredients together and stir thoroughly. Pour the mixture into an ice cube or popsicle tray. Freeze until solid (at least 4 hours).

Note: Make these even more fun by inserting your dog's favorite biscuit or chew into each well of the ice cube tray. A treat inside a treat? Now that's a party.

FROSTY PEANUT BUTTER PUMPKIN FILLER

{ KEEP YOUR DOG BUSY FOR HOURS WITH THIS TASTY FROZEN TREAT }

½ c. peanut butter (unsalted, natural)
½ c. pureed pumpkin (canned or fresh)
2 c. plain nonfat yogurt
CBD oil (see page 16 for dosage amounts)

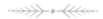

Combine all ingredients together and stir thoroughly. Pour the mixture into a hollow plastic chew toy or marrow bone. Freeze until solid (at least 4 hours).

Note: This is a great one to give your dog when you leave and put them in their crate. Or if you're having company over and want to keep your dog busy. It's healthy, and they'll love you for it.

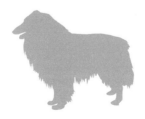

RESOURCES

There are thousands of websites of interest to dog owners these days, and the number of books on natural care continues to grow too (how fortunate for us and our dogs!). We've been to quite a few sites and read lots of books, and this is our list of recommendations.

{ BOOKS ON NUTRITION }

Holistic Guide for a Healthy Dog, by Wendy Volhard and Kerry Brown (Howell Book House, 2000)

Dr. Pitcairn's Complete Guide to Natural Health for Dogs & Cats, by Richard H. Pitcairn, DVM, PhD, and Susan Hubble Pitcairn (Rodale Press, 2005)

The Goldsteins' Wellness & Longevity Program: Natural Care for Dogs and Cats, by Robert S. Goldstein, VMD, and Susan J. Goldstein (TFH Publications, 2005)

{ INTERNET REFERENCE SITES }

www.pawcbd.com

www.aspca.org
A wealth of information, including a list of substances that are poisonous to animals.

https://vet.library.cornell.edu/free-animal-health-resources/
A reliable network of informative websites and articles on all aspects of animal care, nutrition, behavior, disease, and so on.

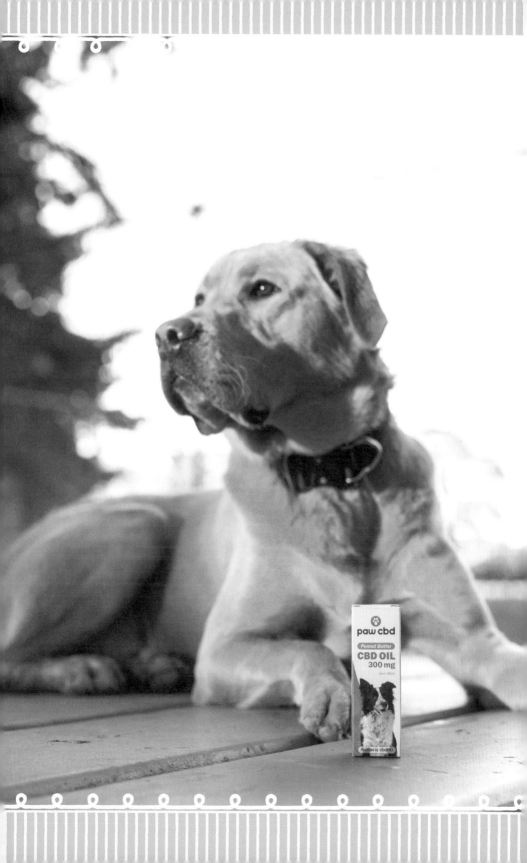

RECIPE INDEX

{ ABOUT PAW CBD BY cbdMD }

Paw CBD is the pet division of cbdMD, one of the most recognized and trusted CBD wellness brands in the world. Paw CBD takes a science-based approach to product development, with a robust testing program and GMP-certified facilities to make innovative CBD products for people and pets.

The patent-pending Superior Broad Spectrum formula by cbdMD and Paw CBD is free of detectable THC and standardizes CBD, CBG, CBN, and terpene levels across all product batches. This means every product is made to the highest safety standards to deliver the ideal balance for the comfort and care of pets. Paw CBD has also earned the National Animal Supplement Council (NASC) Quality Seal, which requires adhering to strict quality standards, meeting label claims, and passing an independent audit to ensure compliance with rigorous quality system requirements.

Paw CBD products are specially formulated with tempting flavors and in milligram strengths based on your pet's weight to help you find the right option to suit their needs and lifestyle. In addition to CBD oil tinctures, treats, peanut butter, and topicals, Paw CBD also offers specialty formulas like Calming, Hip+Joint, and Kidney Support to help address specific wellness issues.

Our pets mean the world to us, and finding ways to help them live better lives is always a priority. Whether you share your life with a pampered pooch or a fabulous feline (or both!), you want them to be healthy and happy, so you make sure they get all the care, love, and exercise they need. You want safe, pet-friendly wellness options you can trust. Paw CBD is a perfect choice–especially if you're looking for a more natural alternative free of added chemicals, fillers, and unnecessary ingredients.

The Paw CBD mission is simple: Make the very best CBD oil to help unleash every pet's potential.

- Specially formulated for pets
- THC free*
- No added fillers or artificial ingredients
- Superior Broad Spectrum CBD oil
- CBD sourced from US hemp
- Third-party, ISO-certified lab tested
- Multiple strengths, formulas, and flavors
- National Animal Supplement Council Quality Seal (tinctures, chews)

{ PAW CBD OIL }

If you are interested in using Paw CBD oil tinctures in your dog treat recipes, visit pawcbd.com to see all the options available. We also have a CBD peanut butter perfect for using in homemade dog treats.

THC free is defined as below the level of detection using validated scientific methods.

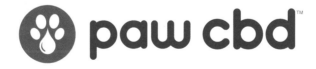

VISIT US AT www.pawcbd.com

{ ABOUT CIDER MILL PRESS }

Good ideas ripen with time. From seed to harvest, Cider Mill Press brings fine reading, information, and entertainment together between the covers of its creatively crafted books. Our Cider Mill bears fruit twice a year, publishing a new crop of titles each spring and fall.

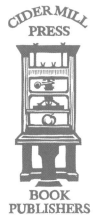

CIDER MILL
PRESS

BOOK
PUBLISHERS

Where good books
are ready for press

VISIT US ONLINE
cidermillpress.com

OR WRITE TO US AT
PO Box 454
Kennebunkport, Maine 04046